Essays in the Economics of
Health and Medical Care

NATIONAL BUREAU OF ECONOMIC RESEARCH

*Human Behavior
and Social Institutions 1*

Essays in the Economics of Health and Medical Care

Edited by
VICTOR R. FUCHS
The City University of New York

NATIONAL BUREAU OF
ECONOMIC RESEARCH
New York 1972

Distributed by Columbia University Press
New York and London

ISBN: 0–87014–236–4

Printed in the United States of America

To the memory of George James, M.D.,
a pioneer in the application of
social science to the
advancement of health

Contents

PART III: THE PRODUCTION OF HEALTH

PART IV: SPATIAL VARIATIONS
IN MORTALITY RATES

Tables

Charts

Figures

Acknowledgments

The initial funding for the NBER program of research in the economics of health was provided by the Commonwealth Fund. The encouragement and support of the Fund and its president, Quigg Newton, were particularly valuable, coming as they did at a time when the problems of health economics were not as widely recognized as they are today. The principal support for the program has been provided by the National Center for Health Services Research and Development, Department of Health, Education, and Welfare (grant 2 Pol HS 00451-04).

A multidisciplinary advisory committee, originally under the chairmanship of the late Dr. George James and currently under that of Dr. Kurt Deuschle, has provided valuable guidance. Other members of the committee, past and present, include Gary S. Becker, Morton Bogdonoff, M.D., James Brindle, Norton Brown, M.D., Eveline Burns, Philip E. Enterline, Marion B. Folsom, Eli Ginzberg, William Gorham, Richard Kessler, M.D., the late David Lyall, M.D., Jacob Mincer, Melvin Reder, Peter Rogatz, M.D., James Strickler, M.D., and Gus Tyler. I would also like to record my gratitude to Rufus Rorem, who first exposed me to the problems in this field, and to the NBER directors who reviewed this manuscript—Moses Abramovitz, Joseph Beirne, and Willard Thorp. The latter's comments were particularly helpful.

The program has been served by an able group of research assistants, including Carol Breckner, Bonnie Garrett, Phyllis Goldberg, Eugene Lewit, Robert Linn, Dimitri Mavros, Elizabeth Rand, Deborah Sarachek, and Ira Silver. Secretarial and typing assistance has been provided by Kay Barthelmes, Terry Battipaglia, Maria Perides, Susanne Kaufman, and Lorraine Lusardi. It is also a pleasure to thank Charlotte Boschan and her staff for programing assistance, Elizabeth Rand, Gnomi Gouldin, and Hedy D. Jellinek for editorial assistance, and H. Irving Forman for the charts and figures. In addition to these general acknowledgments, certain specific ones are indicated in individual papers.

Introduction

This book appears at a time of mounting public concern over the state of health and the system of medical care in the United States. Federal, state, and local governments find themselves overwhelmed by the rapid rise in the cost of this important service. Because of financial, racial, and geographical barriers, many Americans either obtain no care or obtain it under conditions that are degrading and inimical to good care; some patients experience shortages of personnel and facilities even when they are willing and able to pay the going price. In many quarters there is increasing awareness that the United States compares unfavorably with many developed countries with respect to such important health indexes as infant mortality and life expectancy; and within the medical profession itself questions are being raised about medical education, research, and practice.

Interest in the economic aspects of health problems is particularly strong. The National Bureau began a program of research in this field a few years ago, anticipating that our work might be relevant to decision makers some day. That day has come sooner than expected. Increasingly, economists are being called upon for advice concerning the determinants of the utilization of medical care, the efficiency with which resources are used in this industry, the value of improvements in health, the appropriateness of medical care prices and wages, and the creation of new devices for financing medical care. As a result, my colleagues and I have had to divide our time between the slow accumulation of reliable measures and analyses, on the one hand, and the discussion of current problems and preliminary conclusions with physicians, government officials, and other groups with strong policy concerns, on the other. This book reflects these diverse demands. The essays it contains (many of which have appeared previously in highly specialized journals)—along with related NBER studies by Michael Grossman ("The Demand for Health: A Theoretical and Empirical Investigation") and Marcia Kramer and me ("Determinants of Expenditures for Physicians' Services in the United States") to be published shortly—should be viewed as interim reports on a continuing program of research by the National Bureau.

This program has two major objectives. First, we are trying to gain some insights into the factors that determine health levels in the United States. In particular, we are concerned with estimating the relative contributions of medical care and numerous socioeconomic variables, such as income and schooling. From the outset we have found it important to distinguish between health and medical care. This distinction is given its fullest theoretical treatment in Grossman's study, but it is implicit in all our work. Our second principal focus is on the determinants of the cost of medical care and the two components of this cost—utilization and unit price. This concern has led us to consideration of the demand for medical care and the organization of the medical care industry. In addition to our research objectives, we have sought to establish a link between health experts who are unaware of economics and economists who are relatively unfamiliar with a sector that now accounts for over seven per cent of the gross national product.

A brief introduction to each of the essays in this volume is in order. The papers in Part I are intended primarily for physicians and other health specialists. They delineate the concepts, definitions, and methods used by economists in approaching problems of health and medical care. For economists, they may serve as an introduction to some of the institutional peculiarities and policy problems encountered in this sector. The first paper (chapter 1) indicates the relevance of economics to health—namely, that in a world of scarce resources and competing wants choices have to be made, indeed are being made, with regard to the amount and distribution of health services. The economist's role is to help rationalize the decision-making process so that society may best satisfy its objectives with respect to health and other goals. The paper also considers some of the special characteristics of the health industry, such as the high costs of information, the barriers to competition, and the widespread view that services should be related to need rather than ability to pay. It raises, but by no means solves, the problems of how to measure health and how to measure the contribution of health services to health. (These questions receive more systematic attention in the studies by Auster, Leveson, and Sarachek, by Silver, and by Grossman.) Another theme introduced in the first paper which reappears in several others that follow is the significance of individual behavior in determining health. Decisions concerning diet, smoking, exercise, and the like may have more effect on morbidity and mortality than does the consumption of medical care.

The second paper (chapter 2) sets out the traditional economic concepts of demand and supply, and asks how these concepts might be applied to explain the rapid increase in health care's share of the gross national product (from under 4 per cent in 1929 to 5.5 per cent in 1960 and to 7 per cent in 1970). The most important reason seems to be a rise in the price of health services relative to other prices facing a relatively inelastic demand. Other factors mentioned include the growth of third-party payment, a shift from household to market production of health services (e.g., nursing homes for the aged), the introduction of radically new medical procedures, and the possible need for more medical care to offset adverse changes in the environment and life-style.[1] (Some of these matters receive more systematic attention in K. K. Ro's paper in Part II, p. 69, and in V. Fuchs and M. Kramer, "Determinants of Expenditures for Physicians' Services in the United States," NBER, forthcoming.)

The final essay in Part I (chapter 3) discusses three widely shared objectives for the health care system—increasing effectiveness, efficiency, and equity. An effort is made to clarify these objectives and to indicate some of the obstacles to their realization. Reference is made to the possible surplus of surgeons, a subject now receiving major attention at the National Bureau.[2]

Chapter 4, the first essay in Part II, returns to the question raised in chapter 2—Why have medical care expenditures risen so rapidly in recent decades? The hypothesis that the physician plays a major role in determining the demand for care is introduced.[3] It is also argued that the physician's decisions are heavily influenced by a "technological imperative"—the desire to give all the care technically possible without regard to balancing potential benefit against potential cost. The implication of this behavior for the allocation of resources is discussed.

[1] On this last point see Auster, Leveson, and Sarachek, pp. 153–58 below.

[2] See Hughes, Fuchs, Jacoby, and Lewit, "Surgical Workloads in a Community Practice," *Surgery,* March, 1972, for the fist study in this NBER project.

[3] Some support for this hypothesis is found in Fuchs and Kramer, "Determinants of Expenditures for Physicians' Services in the United States," NBER, forthcoming.

Kong-Kyun Ro's study of hospital utilization (chapter 5), which follows, suggests that utilization is not entirely governed by technological considerations. The author examines the length of stay, number of services received, and size of hospital bill for 9,000 patients discharged from twenty-two short-term general hospitals in the Pittsburgh area. After adjusting for diagnostic category, significant differences in utilization are found, depending upon who pays the major portion of the hospital bill. Patients who pay directly have the shortest stays and the smallest bills. Patients whose bills are paid by government have the longest stays and largest bills. Patients covered by insurance have intermediate utilization. This study also shows significant relationships between hospital characteristics and utilization. The presence of teaching programs in a hospital, for instance, is shown to increase the amount of care provided to patients with given diseases.

An entirely different analysis of variations in health care is provided by Morris Silver in the third paper of Part II (chapter 6). He combines unpublished data from the National Center For Health Statistics with information from the 1/1,000 sample of the 1960 *Census of Population* to explain differences in medical care expenditures and work-loss rates across twenty-four region-age-sex groups. Major attention is given to the estimation of income elasticities, and the results indicate an over-all elasticity (with respect to expenditures) of 1.2, with individual components ranging from 0.85 for physicians' services to over 2.0 for dental expenditures.

Part II concludes with a comparison of the distribution of earnings in health and other industries. As noted earlier (chapter 4), there is a continuum of need for medical care, ranging from very simple supportive services to the most complex diagnostic and therapeutic procedures. One might expect a continuum of health service personnel to meet this need, but the paper by Rand, Garrett, and me (chapter 7) shows that most persons in the health industry earn either less than the industry mean or more than twice the industry mean. In comparison with other industries there is a marked absence of personnel in the middle professional and supervisory range. To our surprise, this gap appears to be equally present in the manpower structure of a large, comprehensive, prepaid group practice plan. We suggest that this may be related to the licensure laws and other legislative or professional restrictions on the deployment of health manpower.

The study by Auster, Leveson, and Sarachek in Part III (chapter 8) is a pioneering attempt to measure the impact of medical care and other variables on health. They use statewide data and measure health by age-adjusted mortality. Inputs of medical care are measured alternatively by expenditures or by per capita numbers of hospital beds, physicians, and other medical personnel. Alternative models and estimating techniques all yield similar conclusions, namely, that at the margin the reduction in mortality attributable to additional medical care is small. A 1 per cent increase in medical care appears to be associated with a 0.1 per cent decrease in mortality. The partial association between health and schooling is much stronger. When other variables are held constant, income is found to be positively related to mortality.[4]

The authors suggest that this may be related to the consumption habits associated with higher incomes, or reflect the adverse effects on health of earning a higher income. Such a view would help to explain why age-adjusted death rates remained relatively constant in the United States between 1955 and 1965, in spite of a substantial increase in the per capita quantity of medical services and advances in medical science.

The paper by Auster, Leveson, and Sarachek deals only with the U.S. white population. In the final part of this book (chapter 9), Silver examines similar questions, but from a different point of view and with special attention to black-white differentials in mortality. He uses data for standard metropolitan statistical areas as well as states, studies males and females separately, examines the effect of the source of income (labor or nonlabor) on the relationship with mortality, and introduces a large number of other variables intended to measure various environmental and life-style factors that may influence health.

Silver also finds a strong negative relationship between mortality and schooling. With schooling excluded from the regressions, he finds a negative relation between income and mortality, except for white males across states. The decomposition of income into labor and nonlabor components suggests that the unfavorable aspects of a high income for health may be primarily related to what is involved in earning a high income rather than to consumption patterns. Marital status is another variable that shows significant results. The inverse relationship between mortality and the per cent married with spouse present is particularly strong for black males. A substantial portion of the black-white difference in mortality is explained by the variables examined by the author, but a substantial portion remains unexplained.

Silver carefully notes the qualifications that must be attached to his

[4] Grossman, in his "Demand for Health," reports similar findings, using observations on individuals and measuring health by work-loss days and by self-evaluation of health status.

study—and these apply to all of the conclusions presented in this volume as well. The paucity of data is severe. The quality of the limited data available is often poor, and the conceptual problems are considerable. We regard our findings primarily as hypotheses that require further testing and we are currently attempting to do this in a number of related projects.[5]

VICTOR R. FUCHS

[5] Some of the subjects now under study at the National Bureau are hospital behavior (Barry Chiswick); the correlation between health and schooling (Michael Grossman); the utilization of surgical manpower (Edward F. X. Hughes); the demand for abortion (Marcia Kramer); accidents (William Landes); infant mortality (Eugene Lewit); and malpractice (Melvin Reder).

Essays in the Economics of
Health and Medical Care

PART I

AN ECONOMIST'S VIEW OF HEALTH AND MEDICAL CARE

1

The Contribution of Health Services to the American Economy   *Victor R. Fuchs*

INTRODUCTION

Good health is one of man's most precious assets. The desire to live, to be well, to maintain full command over one's faculties, and to see one's loved ones free from disease, disability, or premature death are among the most strongly rooted of all human desires. That is particularly true of Americans, who, on the whole, eschew the fatalism or preoccupation with the hereafter that is characteristic of some other cultures.

These sentiments are widely held. Therefore, is not the question— "What is the contribution of health services to the United States economy?"—presumptuous? Who can place a value on a life saved, on a body spared from pain, or on a mind restored to sanity? If not presumptuous, is not the question a foolish one, and likely to evoke an equally foolish answer?

When an economist enters an area such as health—so tinged with emotion, so enveloped in an esoteric technology and vocabulary—he runs a high risk of being either irrelevant or wrong. What, then, is the justification for such an inquiry? The principal one is the fact that the question of the contribution of health services is being asked and answered every day. It is being asked and answered implicity every time consumers, hospitals, universities, business firms, foundations, government agencies, and legislative bodies make decisions concerning

NOTE: This article has appeared in the *Milbank Memorial Fund Quarterly*, 44, Part 2, October 1966, pp. 65–101.

I am grateful to Deborah W. Sarachek for the preparation of the bibliography and tables and for numerous contributions to the text. I am also grateful to Dr. Richard H. Kessler for reading the section on medical care, and to Irving Leveson for several useful suggestions.

the volume and composition of health services, present and future. If economists can help to rationalize and make more explicit the decision-making process, provide useful definitions, concepts and analytical tools, and develop appropriate bodies of data and summary measures, they will be making a contribution of their own to health and to the economy.

Plan of the Paper

This paper has limited objectives. It does not pretend to offer a measure of the contribution of health services. Even partial completion of such a task would require a major effort by a research team over a period of several years. Statistics are presented, but for illustrative purposes only.

My primary purpose here is to set out in nontechnical terms how the problem looks to an economist, to discuss definitions, concepts, and methods of measurement, to indicate sources of information, and to suggest promising research approaches. The paper offers a highly personal view of the problem rather than a synthesis of all points of view. Some discussion of relevant literature is included, but no attempt has been made to be exhaustive. Moreover, the scope is limited to the assigned topic and does not provide a general review of the health economics literature. An over-all survey of the field, through 1964, is available in Klarman [26]. In addition, useful bibliographies may be found in Mushkin [44], Wolf [79], and the proceedings of a 1962 conference at the University of Michigan on the economics of health and medical care [76].

First this paper will consider the meaning of "contribution." Then it will go on to discuss the inputs to health services, the outputs of health services (with special emphasis on health), and the contribution of health to the economy. It concludes with a brief summary and suggestions for research.

THE CONCEPT OF CONTRIBUTION

One frequently reads discussions of the contribution of an industry couched in terms of the number of jobs it provides, the volume of its capital investment, and the value of its purchases from suppliers. Such use of the term is ill-advised.

In economic terms the contribution of an industry to the economy should be measured in terms of its output (what does it provide for the economy?), not in terms of its input (what drains does it make on the available supply of resources?). The fundamental fact of economic life is that resources are scarce relative to human wants. Despite a great deal of loose talk about automation and cybernetics, the desires for goods and services in this country and the world exceed the available supplies. Indeed, if this were not the case, no reason could be found to study the economics of health or the economics of anything else. Additional resources would be devoted to health up to the point where no health want would be unmet. That this cannot be done at present is obvious. The reason should be equally obvious. To devote more resources to health services, the people must be willing to forego some other good or service. To the extent of the unused capacity in the economy, some increase could be obtained without diversion from other ends. The extent of this unused capacity, however, relative to the total economy, is very small at the present time.

What is the output of the health industry? No completely satisfactory answer is available. One possible way to think about the problem is to distinguish three different kinds of output that flow from health services. They are health, validation services, and other consumer services.

Probably the most important of these, and certainly the one that has received the most attention, is the contribution of health services to health. However, to define the output of the health industry in terms of some ultimate utility, such as health rather than health services, runs counter to the general practice followed by economists in the study of other industries. For the most part, economists follow the dictum, "whatever Lola gets, Lola wants." They assume that consumers know what they want and know how to satisfy these wants. They further assume that goods and services produced under competitive conditions will be sold at a price which properly reflects (at the margin) the cost of production and the value to the consumer. The health industry, however, has certain characteristics, discussed by Arrow [8], Klarman [26], and Mushkin [45], which suggest that special treatment is required. In the present context, three important differences could be emphasized between the health industry and the "typical" or "average" industry.

Consumer Ignorance

Although expenditures for health services account for more than 6 per cent of all personal consumption expenditures, consumers are, for the most part, terribly ignorant about what they are buying. Very few industries could be named where the consumer is so dependent upon the producer for information concerning the quality of the product. In the typical case he is even subject to the producer's recommendation concerning the quantity to be purchased. A recent report by the American Medical Association says flatly, "The 'quantity' of the hospital services consumed in 1962 was determined by physicians [4, vol. 1, p. 19]."

The question is even more complicated, as indicated in the following statement by J. Douglas Colman, president of the New York Blue Cross [5]:

We must remember that most elements of hospital and medical care costs are generated by or based on professional medical judgment. These judgments include the decision to admit and discharge patients, the decision to order the various diagnostic or therapeutic procedures for patients, and the larger decision as to the types of facilities and services needed by an institution for proper patient care. For the most part, these professional judgments are rendered outside of any organizational structure that fixes accountability for the economic consequences of these judgments.

One reason for consumer ignorance is the inherent uncertainty of the effect of the service on any individual. How can the lay person be expected to know the value of a particular procedure or treatment, when in many cases the medical profession itself is far from agreed? Also, many medical services are infrequently purchased. The average consumer will buy many more automobiles during a lifetime than he will major operations. Therefore, he cannot develop the necessary expertise. Furthermore, the consumer is often not in a good position to make a cool, rational judgment at the time of purchase because he is ill, or because a close member of his family is ill. Finally, the profession does little to inform the consumer; in fact, it frequently takes positive action to keep him uninformed. This leads to the second important difference.

Restrictions on Competition

In some other industries where the possibilities for consumer ignorance are considerable, the consumer obtains protection through the competitive behavior of producers. If the producers are engaged in vigorous competition with one another, some of them, at least, will go out of their way to inform the consumer about the merits of their product and those of the competition. Also, middlemen, such as retailers, are usually involved, one of whose main functions is to provide information and dispel consumer ignorance. In the case of physicians' services (and this is the keystone to health services because of the dominant role of the physician in the industry) the reverse is true. In the first place, severe restrictions on entry are assured through the medical profession's control of medical schools, licensing requirements, and hospital appointments. Advertising is forbidden and price competition is severely frowned upon. Critical comment concerning the output of other physicians is also regarded as unethical.

A good example of the conflict and confusion on this point can be found in the AMA report previously cited. First an extensive discussion of medical care in America is presented, and an attempt is made to identify it with the competitive free enterprise system. The report then goes on to say, "The Medical Care Industry has as its prime social goal the development and maintenance of optimum health levels [4, vol. 1, p. 9]." The authors apparently fail to realize the inconsistency of this statement with their attempt to place the industry in the context of a market system. In such a system, industries do not have "social goals." The goal of the individual firm is maximum profit (or minimum loss); the achievement of social goals is a by-product of the profit-seeking activities of individual firms and industries.

Numerous arguments can be advanced in support of each of the restrictive practices followed by the medical profession. (Arrow's discussion [8] of the role of uncertainty in health is particularly relevant.) In the present context, these restrictive practices mean that an appraisal of the industry's output and performance by economists cannot be pursued using the same assumptions that would be appropriate in appraising the output of a more competitive industry.

The Role of "Need"

Health services are one of a small group of services which many people believe should be distributed according to need rather than demand (i.e., willingness and ability to pay). Other services in this category, such as education, police and fire protection, and sanitation are typically provided by government. For a time philanthropy and the generosity of physicians were relied upon to achieve this distribution for health services, but now increasing reliance is being placed on taxation or coverage in compulsory insurance schemes. If "need" is to be the criterion, however, a closer examination of the role of health services in filling that need seems in order.

If a person "demands" an article of clothing or a haircut or some other good or service, in the sense of being willing and able to pay for it, usually no special cause for concern or inquiry arises on the part of anyone else regarding either the need underlying the demand or whether the purchase will satisfy the need. However, if a service, such as health, is to be provided to others on the basis of "need," then those paying for it would seem to have some right to inquire into the actual presence of "need," and an obligation to determine whether or how much the service actually satisfies the need. Because need is often the criterion for obtaining health services, much of the payment for these services is by a "third party." This means that the consumer has less incentive to make certain that the output (what he is getting) is truly worth the cost.

These characteristics of the health industry indicate why output cannot simply be equated with expenditures. However, that does not mean that economic analysis cannot be applied to this industry. On the contrary, precisely these special characteristics make the industry an interesting subject for economic analysis, both from the scientific and public policy points of view.

Total Versus Marginal Contribution

In studying the contribution of health services to health, the *total* contribution must be distinguished from the *marginal* contribution. The total contribution can be appraised by asking what would happen if no health services at all were available. The results would almost surely be disastrous in terms of health and life expectancy. A reasonably safe conclusion seems to be that the total contribution is enormous. A modern economy could not continue to function without some health services.

The marginal contribution, on the other hand, refers to the effects on health of a small increase or decrease in the amount of health services provided. To expect a small change in services to have a large effect on the level of health is, of course, out of the question. But that is not what is being measured. Rather, the question is, what is the relative effect on health of a small relative change in health services?

The reason this question is crucial is that changes are usually being made at the margin. Most decisions are not of the "all or nothing" variety, but involve "a little more or a little less." The goal of an economic system, in terms of maximum satisfaction, is to allocate resources in such a way that the last (marginal) inputs of resources used for each purpose make contributions that are proportionate to their costs.

HEALTH SERVICES

"Health services" can be defined as services rendered by:
  1. Labor: personnel engaged in medical occupations, such as doc-

tors, dentists, and nurses, plus other personnel working directly under their supervision, such as practical nurses, orderlies, and receptionists.

2. Physical capital: the plant and equipment used by this personnel, e.g., hospitals and x-ray machines.

3. Intermediate goods and services: i.e., drugs, bandages, and purchased laundry services.

This definition corresponds roughly to what economists have in mind when they refer to the "health industry." Payment for this labor, capital, and intermediate input is the basis for estimating "health expenditures."

This definition seems satisfactory for the purposes of this paper, but some classification problems are worth mentioning. First, some health-related resources might or might not be included in health services, such as the provision of a supply of sanitary water. A second problem arises because a portion of the personnel and facilities in hospitals is used to produce "hotel services" rather than health. This paper will not exclude such inputs from health services, but will try to allow for them by showing that part of the output consists of other consumer services (see Figure 1-1 on p. 23).

One of the greatest problems concerns the unpaid health services that people perform for themselves and for members of their families. According to present practice in national income accounting, this labor input is not included in health services. Therefore, this "home" production must be treated as part of the environmental factors that affect health.

Approximately two-thirds of the value of health services in the United States represents labor input. Somewhat less than one-sixth represents input of physical capital, and the remainder represents goods and services purchased from other industries. These are all rough estimates. Information about the volume and composition of health services must be derived from a variety of official and unofficial sources. No census of the health industry compares to the census of manufacturing, trade, or selected services. As the importance of the health industry grows, the government may wish to consider whether a periodic census of health should be undertaken.

Present sources of information are of two main types: those that give information about expenditures for health services and those that report on one or more aspects of inputs of resources. A good example of the former is the material supplied by Reed and Rice [48]. A few problems arise when these data are used to measure inputs of health services. First, some of the items represent investment expenditures by the health industry rather than payment for current services. Expenditures for construction and medical research are the most important ones in this category. No particular economic justification may be found for treating these as inputs in the year that the investment takes place. On the other hand, current input of capital may be understated to the extent that hospital charges do not include an allowance for depreciation and interest.

The expenditures shown for drugs, eyeglasses, etc. do not all represent payment for intermediate goods purchased from other industries. A substantial portion (probably about one-half) represents the labor services of pharmacists, opticians, and the like, and the services of the plant and equipment used by this personnel.

The net cost of health insurance represents output of the insurance industry. It may be thought of as an intermediate service purchased and resold by the health industry.

A final point concerns the failure of expenditures data to reflect contributed labor. This results in an underestimate of labor input, especially in hospitals.

Other sources of information on expenditures for health services include: the Office of Business Economics [67, 68, 69], detailed annual data on personal consumption expenditures for health services; the Social Security Administration [41], special emphasis on government spending for health services; the Public Health Service [71, 72], expenditures cross-classified with characteristics of the individual incurring the expense; the Health Information Foundation [6]; and the Bureau of Labor Statistics [62, 63].

The decennial population census [65] is an excellent source of information about labor inputs to health services. In addition to providing a complete enumeration of the number employed and their geographical location, numerous economic and demographic characteristics are described in considerable detail. With the aid of the 1/1000 sample of the 1960 census [66], comparisons may be made within the health industry and between health and other industries on such matters as education, earnings, age, sex, race, and hours of work. The labor input to health services may be defined as all persons employed in the health and hospital industry, plus those persons in medical occupations employed in other industries. Health employment, so defined, amounted to almost three million in 1960. This represented almost 5 per cent of total employment.

Another good source of data on labor input is provided by the Public Health Service [74]. This source is particularly useful for those interested in such characteristics as physicians' type of practice, specialization, medical school, and location of practice.

Information on capital inputs to health services is more difficult to obtain. The annual guide book of *Hospitals* reports the book value of hospital plant and equipment [3]. This was given as 21.3 billion dollars in 1963. This figure is biased downward as a measure of present value because of the rise in prices of construction in recent decades. It is biased upward to the extent that hospitals have failed to make deductions for depreciation. This same source also provides useful data on labor input by type and size of hospital.

Some information on the capital inputs associated with the labor input of physicians can be gleaned from the reports of the United States Internal Revenue Service [75]. According to these reports, 163,000 returns were filed for unincorporated businesses under the heading of "physicians, surgeons, and oculists" in 1962. These returns showed business receipts of six billion dollars. They showed net rent paid of 250 million dollars (most of this represents payment for capital services) as well as depreciation charges of 190 million dollars. Some information for other types of health services, such as those provided by dentists and dental surgeons, is also available from the same source.

One important source of information about inputs of equipment and intermediate goods that has not received much attention is the quinquennial Census of Manufactures [64]. The latest one provides considerable data on shipments by manufacturers of drugs, ophthalmic goods, dental equipment and supplies, ambulances, hospital beds, and many other health items.

Real Versus Money Costs

One problem in measuring inputs that has already been alluded to in connection with volunteer labor is the need to distinguish between "real" and "money" costs. The person who is not an economist usually thinks of the cost of health services in money terms; when more money has to be spent, costs are said to be rising. This approach is readily understandable and for some purposes useful and proper. The analysis of many problems, however, requires a stripping away of the money veil and an examination of "real" costs. The real cost to society of providing health services, or any other good or service, consists of the labor and capital used in the industry, plus the cost of producing the intermediate goods and services. For instance, if the workers employed in a given hospital are unionized, and they negotiate a large increase in wages, the money costs of that hospital clearly rise, other factors remaining unchanged. But the real cost of that hospital service has not changed at all.

In a perfectly competitive market economy, money costs usually provide a good measure of real costs. But in the health industry, with its curious mixture of philanthropy, government subsidies, imperfect labor markets, and contributed labor time, concentration on money costs alone may frequently be misleading. Good decisions about the allocation of resources require information about the real costs involved.

One important element of real cost is often overlooked, namely, the time of the patient. When the patient is ill, the value of this time (measured by alternative opportunities) may be very low. But, in calculating the costs of periodic medical examinations and routine visits, omitting this cost would be a mistake [9].

HEALTH SERVICES AND HEALTH

Any attempt to analyze the relationship between health services and health runs headlong into two very difficult problems. The first concerns the definition and measurement of levels of health, or at least changes in levels. The second involves an attempt to estimate what portion of changes in health can be attributed to health services, as distinct from the genetic and environmental factors that also affect health. Therefore, the question of definition and measurement of health levels is next on the agenda, while the second problem is examined below.

What is Health?

Definitions of health abound. Agreement is hard to find. The oft-quoted statement of the World Health Organization [80] is framed in positive (some would say Utopian) terms: "A state of complete physical and mental and social well-being." Others, e.g., Ffrangcon Roberts [49], simply stress the absence of, or the ability to resist, disease and death.

A few points seem clear. First, health has many dimensions—anatomical, physiological, mental, and so on. Second, the relative importance of different disabilities varies considerably, depending upon the particular culture and the role of the particular individual in that culture. Third, most attempts at measurement take the negative approach. That is, they make inferences about health by measuring the degree of ill health, as indicated by mortality, morbidity, disability, et cetera. Finally, with respect to health, as in so many other cases, detecting changes in health is easier than defining or measuring absolute levels.

Indexes of Health

The most widely used indicators of health levels are those based on mortality rates, either age-specific or age-adjusted. The great virtues of death rates are that they are determined objectively, are readily available in considerable detail for most countries, and are reasonably comparable for intertemporal and interspatial comparisons.

Health experts rely heavily on mortality comparisons for making judgments about the relative health levels of whites and nonwhites in the United States, or of smokers versus nonsmokers, and for other problems. A recent survey of health in Israel [23], for example, concluded:

The success of the whole system of medicine in Israel is best judged, not by an individual inspection of buildings or asking the opinions of doctors and patients, but by an examination of the health statistics of the country. Infant mortality is about the same as in many European countries, and life expectancy is equal to, or better than, most.

The tendency in recent years has been to dismiss mortality as a useful indicator of health levels in developed countries because very little intranational or international variation occurs. These reports of the demise of mortality indexes are premature.

Differences within the United States are still considerable. The most important differential is race, but even considering rates for whites only, the age-adjusted death rate (average 1959–61) in the highest state is 33 per cent greater than in the lowest; the highest infant mortality rate is 55 per cent above the lowest; and the death rate for males 45–54 in the worst state is 60 per cent higher than in the state with the lowest rate.

Comparing the United States with other developed countries, the differences are even more striking, as shown in Table 1-1. For males 45–54 (a critical age group from the point of view of production), the United States has the highest rate of any country in the Organization for Economic Cooperation and Development (OECD), a rate which is almost double that of some of the other countries. Such gross differences surely present a sufficient challenge for scientific analysis and for public policy.

Another argument that seems to underlie the objections to mortality indexes is that age-adjusted death rates (and average life expectancy)

TABLE 1-1

Indexes of Death Rates in OECD Countries Relative to the United States,
Average 1959–61

Country	Age-adjusted Death Rate[a]	Infant Mortality	Mortality Males 45–54	Mortality Females 45–54
United States	100	100	100	100
White	96	88	94	87
Nonwhite	138	164	155	220
Iceland	78	62[c]	62	81
Netherlands	82	63	57	65
Norway	82	74[c]	54	58
Sweden	86	63	52	69
Greece	86	155	56	64
Denmark	90	85[c]	59	78
Canada	92	107	76	79
Switzerland	94	83	67	75
France	96	105	89	83
Italy	98	166	74	77
Belgium	102	113	82	79
United Kingdom	103	87	76	85
Spain	104[b]	178	75[b]	84[b]
West Germany (excluding Berlin)	107	129	77	84
Luxembourg	107	122	96	89
Ireland	109	118	74	105
Austria	110	142	87	87
Japan	115	127[c]	83	102
Portugal	131	328	84	84

Sources: For age-adjusted death rate, mortality males 45–54 and mortality females 45–54, see, for the United States, U.S. Public Health Service, *Vital Statistics of the United States, 1959, 1960, 1961* (deaths), and U.S. Bureau of the Census, *1960 Census of Population, Volume 1, Characteristics of the Population*, Part 1, United States Summary (population). For OECD Countries, see World Health Organization, *Annual Epidemiological and Vital Statistics, 1959, 1960, 1961*. Data for Luxembourg are from United Nations, *Demographic Yearbook, 1960, 1961.*

For infant mortality rate, see United Nations, *Demographic Yearbook, 1961*, Table 17.

[a] Age-adjustment is by the "indirect" method. For each country, U.S. age-specific death rates were applied to the actual population distribution and the result was divided into the actual number of deaths to obtain the mortality ratio, i.e., the age-adjusted death rate in index number form.

[b] 1957–59 average.

[c] 1958–60 average.

have been relatively stable in the United States for the past decade. The real costs of health services have increased over this period, and medical science has certainly made some progress; therefore, one may assume that some improvement in health levels occurred that was not captured by the mortality indexes.

This type of reasoning begs the question. Possibly the increase in health services has not resulted in improved health levels and the scientific advances of recent years have not had much effect on health. An alternative explanation is that changes in environmental factors in these years have had, on balance, a negative effect on health, thus offsetting the favorable effects of increases in services and medical knowledge. The latter explanation seems to be a very real possibility. Health services do not operate in a vacuum, nor can they be regarded as being matched against a "health destroying nature" that remains constant over time. An apt aphorism attributed to Sigerist states that "each civilization makes its own diseases [42]."

Most of the suggestions for new and better indexes of health involve combining morbidity and mortality information. An excellent discussion of some of the problems to be encountered, and possible solutions, may be found in Sullivan [58]. One particularly intriguing approach, suggested by Sanders [52], consists in calculating years of "effective" life expectancy, based on mortality and morbidity rates. Such an index would measure the number of years that a person could expect to live and be well enough to fulfill the role appropriate to his sex and age. This approach could be modified to take account of the fact that illness or disability is a matter of degree. The years deducted from life expectancy because of disability should be adjusted by some percentage factor that represents the degree of disability. The determination of these percentage weights is one of the most challenging research problems to be faced in calculating a health index.

The Impact of Health Services on Health

Writing this section would be more appropriate for a physician than for an economist, since the relation between health services and health is a technical question best answered by those whose training is in that technology. All that is intended here is to record some impressions by an outsider who has reviewed a minute portion of the literature from a particular point of view.

The impact of health services on health depends upon two factors: (1) How effective are the best-known techniques of diagnosis, therapy, et cetera? (2) How wide is the gap between the best-known techniques ("treatment of choice") and those actually used across the country? The latter question has been reviewed extensively in medical literature under the heading "quality of care" [7]; it will not be discussed here.

A useful introduction to the first question is provided in Terris [61].

The belief that an important relationship exists between health services and health is of long standing. Reliable evidence to support this belief is of much more recent origin. For thousands of years sick people sought advice and treatment of physicians and surgeons, but many of the most popular remedies and courses of treatment of earlier centuries are now known to have been either harmful or irrelevant.

If this is true, how can one explain the demand for health services that existed in the past? Two possible explanations seem worth noting; they may even continue to have some relevance today. First, doctors probably received a great a deal of credit that properly belonged to nature. The body itself has great healing powers, and most people who successfully consulted physicians would have recovered from or adjusted to their illness without medical intervention. Second, and probably more important, is the intensive need "to do something" that most people have when faced with pain and the possibility of death.

In more recent times, the value of health services for certain illnesses has been established with considerable certainty; but broad areas of doubt and controversy still remain. The following discussion considers a few examples of each type.

Infectious disease is an area where medical services are demonstrably effective. Although the decline of some infectious diseases (e.g., tuberculosis) should be credited in part to environmental changes such as improved sanitation, the important role played by improvements in medical science cannot be downgraded. For many infectious diseases the health service is preventive rather than curative and "one-shot" rather than continuous. Such preventive services do not occupy a large portion of total physician time, but the results should nevertheless be included in the output of the health industry.

Examples of the control of infectious disease through immunization are: diphtheria [51], tetanus [33, 34], and poliomyelitis [4, vol. 3, chap. 4]; chemotherapy is effective in tuberculosis [4, vol. 3, chap. 7] and pneumonia [29]. The decline in mortality from these causes has been dramatic, and some correlation can be observed between changes in the rate of decline and the adoption of specific medical advances. For example, during the fifteen-year period 1935 to 1950, which spanned the introduction and wide use of sulfonamides and penicillin, the United States death rate from influenza and pneumonia fell at a rate of more than 8 per cent per annum; the rate of decline was 2 per cent per annum from 1900 to 1935. In the case of tuberculosis, considerable progress was made throughout this century, but the relative rate of decline in the death rate accelerated appreciably after the adoption of penicillin, streptomycin, and PAS (para-aminosalicylic acid) in the late 1940's, and of isoniazid in the early 1950's.

Even more dramatic examples are the death rate patterns of syphilis and poliomyelitis, where the introduction of new forms of treatment for the former and immunization for the latter were reflected very quickly in precipitous drops in mortality. To be sure, the diseases mentioned have not been eliminated. Partly for sociocultural reasons, the incidence of syphilis has actually increased in recent years. In other cases, modern treatments of choice are losing their effectiveness because of the development of resistant strains of microorganisms.

The situation with respect to the noninfectious diseases is more mixed. Some examples of demonstrable effectiveness are the following: replacement therapy has lessened the impact of diabetes [37], dental caries in children are reduced by fluoridation [53, 81], and medical care has become increasingly successful in treating trauma [18]. The diagnostic value of the Papanicolaou test for cervical cancer is established [24, 17], and the incidence of invasive cancer of this site was reduced in the 1960's, presumably due to medical treatment during the preinvasive stage disclosed by the test. Also effective is the treatment of skin cancer [27].

Less heartening are the reports on other cancer sites. The five-year survival rate for breast cancer (the most common single organ site of malignancy in either sex) is typically about 50 per cent. Moreover, a review of the breast cancer literature found such striking uniformity of results, despite widely differing therapeutic techniques, that the author was prompted to speculate whether such end results record therapeutic triumphs or merely the natural history of the disease [30]. Some writers stress the importance of prompt treatment for cancer; others question whether elimination of delay would dramatically alter survival rates.[1] The problem of delay itself is complex, and not simply attributable to ignorance or lack of access to health services: "Physicians with cancer are just as likely to delay as are laymen [59]."

Heart disease is another major cause of death where the contribution of health services to health leaves much to be desired. Despite the contributions of surgery in correcting congenital and rheumatic cardiac defects [57] and the decline in recurrence rates of rheumatic fever [78],

---

[1] In May 1971 several reports presented at the American Cancer Society's Second National Conference on Breast Cancer indicated that early detection and treatment resulted in considerable improvement in survival rates for women with breast cancer. (See *The New York Times*, May 19, 1971, p. 30.)

apparently no curative treatment has been found for rheumatic fever [2, 28]. The treatment of coronary heart disease is only partially effective [12]. The value of antihypertensive drugs in preventing early death in case of malignant hypertension seems assured, but these drugs may be harmful in nonmalignant hypertension [15].[2] The value of anti-coagulants in reducing complications and mortality with acute myo-cardial infarction has been questioned by recent reports [2, 31].

Definitive therapy is still not available for widespread afflictions such as cerebral vascular disease [13], and rehabilitation results indicate that only the more severely ill may benefit from formal therapy (the others seem to recover spontaneously) [35]. No cure is known for schizo-phrenia. The tranquilizing drugs and shock therapy have had a significant impact in shortening hospital stay, yet they do not seem to lower rehospitalization rates below those achieved with other methods [38].

Health services have always been assumed to be very valuable in connection with pregnancy, but a recent study of prenatal care reveals little relation to prevention of pregnancy complications or prevention of early pregnancy termination, except in uncomplicated pregnancies of thirty weeks' gestation and over [54]. The latter cases do not clarify whether the medical care component of prenatal care, as distinct from nutritional and other components, deserves the credit.

Innovations in health services are not limited to improvements in drugs, surgical techniques, or other technological changes. Research concerning the effects on health of group practice [55, 56], intensive care units [32, 73], and special arrangements for neonatal surgery [19] has yielded encouraging results with respect to these organizational innovations. In other cases, results have been disappointing, e.g., multiple screening [82], periodic medical examination of school chil-dren [83], and cancer control programs differing in duration, intensity, and cost [39].

This very brief review indicates that no simple generalization is possible about the effect of health services on health. Although many health services definitely improve health, in other cases even the best-known techniques may have no effect. This problem of relating input to output is one of the most difficult ones facing economists who try to do research on the health industry. They must gain the support and advice of doctors and public health specialists if they are to make progress in this area.

[2] Research results published in 1970 indicate a much more favorable prospect regarding drug therapy for nonmalignant hypertension.

Environmental Factors and Health

One of the factors contributing to the difficulty in reaching firm conclusions about the relationship between health services and health is the importance of environmental factors. Some environmental changes are biological, involving the appearance and disappearance of bacteria, viruses, and other sources of disease. Many environmental variables are related to economics in one way or another. Some are tied to the production process, e.g., the factors associated with occupation. Others are part of consumption, e.g., diet and recreation. Major attention has frequently been given to income, partly because many other environmental factors tend to be highly correlated with real income, both over time and cross-sectionally. Examples include housing, education, urbanization, drinking, and the use of automobiles.

The prevailing assumption, in some cases with good evidence, has indicated that an increase in real per capita income has favorable implications for health, apart from the fact that it permits an increase in health services. This assumption for the United States at present, except for infant mortality, may reasonably be questioned. This country may have passed the peak with respect to the favorable impact of a rising level of living on health. This is not to say that some favorable elements are not still associated with a higher income, but the many unfavorable ones may outweigh them.[3]

After a period of neglect of environmental factors by medical researchers, the tendency in recent years has been to overemphasize the favorable aspects of rising income levels. For example, the American Medical Association recently stated, "Medical science does not seek major credit for the improvements in the health levels during the past twenty-five years. Certainly, our standards of living and higher educational levels have contributed substantially to the betterment of the health level in the United States [4, vol. 3, p. ix]." Although modesty is becoming, the Association provides no evidence to support this statement, and the chances are good that it is wrong.

Altendorfer [1] was able to show some slight negative association between age-adjusted death rates and income across cities in the United States in 1940, but the adjustment for the effect of color was crude, and no allowance was made for the correlation between health services and income. The question at issue here is the relation between

[3] See "The Production of Health, an Exploratory Study" by Auster, Leveson, and Sarachek below.

income and health, not of the fact that higher income permits a higher rate of utilization of health services.

Some preliminary work suggests that education is indeed favorable to health, but by far the largest share of the credit for improvement in health levels over the past twenty-five years probably should go to what economists call improvements in technology—better drugs, better medical knowledge, better diagnostic techniques, et cetera. Cross-sectional regressions across states, for instance, reveal a positive relation between income and mortality for whites, except in the case of infant mortality.

Death rate patterns in countries where the level of income is far below that of the United States should also cause one to question the level of living argument. In Table 1-2, death rates for five European countries in 1960 are compared with rates for the United States in 1960 and 1925. The latter date was included because, in 1960, these five countries were at a level of real per capita income roughly comparable to that of the United States in 1925 [16].

The table shows that the over-all age-adjusted death rates for the European countries are very similar to those for the United States, and far below the level of the United States in 1925. The European crude rates tend to be higher because of the larger proportion of older people in Europe. Despite this bias, the crude rates for tuberculosis and influenza and pneumonia (two causes where the rise in income levels has been alleged to be particularly important) are also much closer to the United States in 1960 than to the United States in 1925. One explanation worth investigating is that the European countries enjoy a medical technology that is similar to that of the United States in 1960, and that changes in medical technology have been the principal cause of the decrease in the United States death rate from 1925 to 1960.

One possible reason for the effect of income levels on health having been overestimated is that investigators often find a very high correlation between income and the health status of individuals. The tendency has been to assume that the latter was the result of the former, but some recent studies of schizophrenia [43] and bronchitis [40] suggest that the causal relationship may run the other way. Evidence shows that illness causes a deterioration in occupational status (from a skilled job to an unskilled job and from an unskilled job into unemployment). The evidence relates to the decline in occupational status from father to son (where the latter is a victim of the disease) and also within the patient's own history.

Even though research on the relation between health services and

TABLE 1-2

Comparison of 1925 and 1960 U.S. Death Rates with 1960 Rates in Selected
European Countries
(per 100,000 population)

	Age-adjusted Death Rate (All Causes)[a]	Crude Death Rate (All Causes)	Crude Death Rate, Tuberculosis (All Forms)	Crude Death Rate, Influenza and Pneumonia[b]
1925				
United States	1,683.3	1,170.0	84.8	121.7
1960				
United States	945.7	945.7	5.9	32.9
England and Wales	926.8	1,150.2	7.5	70.1
France	926.8	1,136.2	22.1	48.1
West Germany (excluding Berlin)	983.5	1,136.8	16.2	43.8
Netherlands	766.0	762.1	2.8	26.6
Belgium	1,002.4	1,244.7	17.1	36.5

Sources: For 1925 U.S. data, see U.S. Bureau of the Census, *Historical Statistics of the United States*, series B114–128, B129–142, A22–33. For U.S. age-specific death rates in 1960, see U.S. Department of Health, Education and Welfare, Public Health Service, National Vital Statistics Division, *Vital Statistics of the United States, 1960*, Vol. 2, Part A, Table 1-C. For 1960 European data on population distribution, influenza and pneumonia deaths 1959–61, total populations 1959–61, and total deaths 1960 in West Germany and Belgium, see World Health Organization, *Annual Epidemiological and Vital Statistics, 1959, 1960, 1961*, Table 4. Other crude death rates in 1960: United Nations, *Demographic Yearbook, 1961*, Table 17.

[a] Age-adjustment is by the "indirect" method. For each country the U.S. age-specific death rates in 1960 were applied to the actual population distribution and the result was divided into the actual number of deaths to obtain the age-adjusted death rate index. This was multiplied by the U.S. crude death rate in 1960 to obtian the age-adjusted death rate.

[b] 1959–61 average used instead of 1960 rates because of influenza epidemic in 1960.

health would seem to be primarily the responsibility of those with training in medicine and public health, the long experience that economists have had with environmental variables like income, education, and urbanization suggests that a multidisciplinary approach would be most fruitful.

OTHER CONTRIBUTIONS OF HEALTH SERVICES

The effect of health services on health probably represents their most important contribution. However, two other types of output are worth noting—validation services and other consumer services.

Validation Services

One type of output that is not directly related to improvements in health can be traced to the fact that only a physician can provide judgments concerning a person's health status that will be widely accepted by third parties. This type of output is designated "validation services" in Figure 1-1. One familiar example is the life insurance examination. This examination may have some favorable impact on the health of the examinee, but it need not do so and is not undertaken primarily for that purpose. The insurance company simply wants to know about the health status of the person concerned. In obtaining and providing that information, the physician is producing something of value, but it is not health.

Other examples include a physician's testifying in court, providing information in a workmen's compensation case, or executing a death certificate.

The validation role of physicians is probably much broader than in these sharply defined cases. Consider the following situation: A person feels ill; he has various aches, pains, and other symptoms. He complains and looks for sympathy from family, friends, neighbors, and coworkers. He may seek to be relieved from certain responsibilities or to be excused from certain tasks. Doubts may arise in the minds of persons around him. Questions may be asked. Is he really ill? Is he doing all that he can to get well? A visit, or a series of visits, to one or more doctors is indicated. The patient may not have the slightest hope that these visits will help his health, and, indeed, he may be correct. Nevertheless, the service rendered by the physician cannot be said to result in no output. The visit to the doctor is a socially or culturally necessary act. The examination, the diagnosis, and the prognosis are desired by the patient to provide confirmation to those who have doubts about him. Only the professional judgment of a physician can still the doubts and answer the questions.

The validation service type of output should not be confused with another type of problem that arises in measuring the output of health services—namely, that advance knowledge about the effect of health services on health is sometimes difficult to obtain. This problem is similar to the "dry hole" situation in drilling for oil. That is not to say that the work done in drilling dry holes results in no output. Rather, when the drilling operation is viewed in its entirety, some success will be noted as well as some failures. All those who participate in the drilling operation are considered to be sources of the output. Similarly,

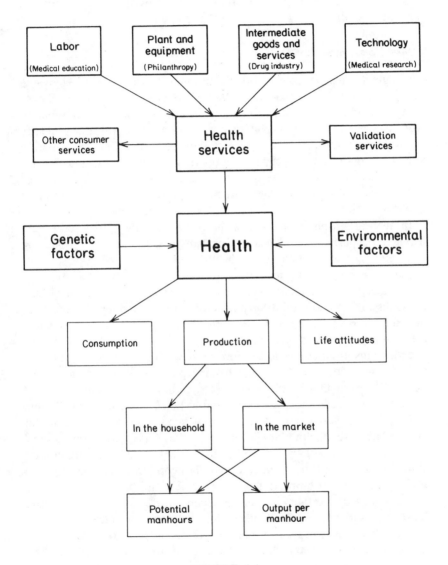

FIGURE 1-1
A Schematic View of the Economics of Health

if a surgeon operates on ten people and only six are helped, one should not say that no output occurred in the other four cases, if one could not determine in advance which cases could be helped and which could not. The output consisted of improving the health of six people, but this output was the result of a production process which encompassed the ten operations.

Other Consumer Services

The outstanding example of other consumer services produced by the health industry is the so-called "hotel" services of hospitals. Those hospital activities that directly affect health are difficult to separate from those that are equivalent to hotel services, but the latter clearly are not insignificant. One way of getting some insight into this question would be to study the occupational distribution of health industry employment. A very significant fraction consists of cooks, chamber maids, porters, and others who are probably producing "other consumer services [48]."

In mental hospitals and other hospitals providing long-term care a major proportion of all costs is probably associated with producing consumer services other than health. The fact that these other consumer services would have to be provided somehow, either publicly or privately, if the patients were not in the hospital is often neglected in discussions of how total hospital costs are inflated by the presence of people who are not really ill. Possibly some of these consumer services are actually produced more inexpensively in a hospital than on the outside. This point comes to the fore in New York City, now grappling with the problem of housing and feeding patients who have been discharged from mental hospitals not because they are cured, but because the new drugs mean they no longer need to be confined to an institution.

Some of the services rendered by nurses outside hospitals also bear little relation to health, but nevertheless they may have considerable value to consumers. This type of service is likely to grow in importance with the increase in the number of elderly people with income who are seeking companionship and help with their daily chores.

The failure of mortality indexes to decline with increased expenditures for health services in recent years has led some people to conclude that mortality no longer measures health levels properly. But if most of these increased expenditures have gone for health services that largely produce "other consumer services" rather than health, a great deal of the mystery is removed.

HEALTH AND THE ECONOMY

An increase in health has two potential values for individuals—consumption and production. Good health is clearly something consumers desire for itself. (That they do not put an overriding value on health is also abundantly clear from the figures on smoking, drinking, overeating, fast driving, et cetera.) To the extent that health services lead to better health, they make a contribution to the economy comparable to that of any industry producing a good or service wanted by consumers.

In addition, better health may contribute to the productive capacity of the economy. It may do this, first, by increasing the supply of potential man-hours through a reduction in mortality and decrease in time lost because of illness and disability. Second, better health may increase production by improving productivity, that is, increasing output per man-hour.

Beyond its potential direct contribution to production and consumption, better health probably has important indirect effects on the economy. These indirect effects occur through the changes in life attitudes which may accompany changes in health. When the average life expectancy in a country is only thirty or thirty-five years, attitudes toward work and saving, for instance, may be different from those in countries where life expectancy is fifty or seventy-five years. When infant mortality rates are very high, attitudes toward birth control are likely to be different from those in countries where mortality rates are low. Indeed, the idea of progress itself may be intimately bound up with the health levels of the population and the rate of change of these levels.

Health and Production

A substantial literature is now available which attempts to measure the impact of changes in health levels on the productive capacity of the economy [26, pp. 162–72]. The principal approach is to ask how many more people are available for work as a result of a decrease in death rates, and what potential or actual production can be attributed to this increased supply of manpower. The capitalized value of the increase at a given point in time can be obtained by summing the value of future potential production represented by the lives saved. Current earnings patterns are usually used with or without adjustment for future increases in earnings per man, and with future earnings discounted at some appropriate interest rate.

The details of calculating the value of lives saved vary greatly from one investigator to another, but one result is common to all: the value

of a man (in terms of future production potential) is very different at
different ages. Table 1-3 shows some calculated values for United
States males at three different discount rates based on average patterns
of earnings and labor force participation rates in 1960.

The principal implication of the age-value profile is that the economic
return (in production terms) from saving a life is not the same at all
ages. Different kinds of health programs and different kinds of medical

TABLE 1-3

Age-Value Profile of United States Males in 1960
Estimated from Discounted Future Earnings

	Discount Rate		
Age	4.0 per Cent per Annum (A)	7.2 per Cent per Annum (B)	10.0 per Cent per Annum (C)
0	$32,518	$14,680	$ 8,114
10	48,133	29,361	21,047
20	68,363	52,717	45,023
30	81,300	70,515	64,697
40	73,057	67,365	64,012
50	54,132	52,406	51,363
60	30,285	29,853	29,570
70	9,395	9,395	9,395
80	2,465	2,465	2,465
90	0	0	0

Note: The indicated discount rates were applied to the following earnings:

Age	Annual Earnings
0–14	$ 0
15–24	1,201
25–34	4,582
35–44	5,569
45–54	5,327
55–64	4,338
65–74	1,386
75–84	493
85 and over	0

No discounting was applied *within* ten-year age groups and no allowance was made
for future increases in real earnings or for life expectancy. Also, no deduction was
made for additional consumption attributable to decreased mortality, and no earnings were imputed for males not in the labor force.

Source: U.S. Bureau of the Census, *1960 Census of Population*, Occupational
Characteristics, Table 34.

research are likely to affect various age groups differently; therefore, wise planning should give some consideration to these matters. For example, accidents accounted for only 6.6 per cent of all male deaths in the United States in 1960, but accounted for 12.8 per cent of the economic cost of these deaths as measured by age-value profile B in Table 1-3. On the other hand, vascular lesions accounted for 9.5 per cent of all male deaths, but only 5.7 per cent of the economic cost of these deaths.

Table 1-4 shows how the age-value profile can be used to calculate the economic value (in production terms only) of the United States, using the 1960 death rate instead of the 1929 rate, or of lowering the United States rate in 1960 to the Swedish rate in 1960. In the former comparison, the greatest savings in number of lives were for infants and ages seventy-five to eighty-four, but the greatest gain from a production point of view was from the reduction in the mortality rate for men thirty-five to forty-four. The United States–Swedish comparison highlights the current importance and potential of the forty-five to fifty-four age group.

Most studies that attempt to place a value on a life saved (or on the cost of premature death) discuss the question of whether some deduction from discounted future earnings should be made for the future consumption of the individuals whose lives are saved. The arguments for and against are usually framed in terms of whether the value being measured is the value to society including the individual or excluding him. A slightly different way of looking at this problem could be suggested. Consider someone contemplating whether a certain expenditure for health services is worthwhile for him in terms of its expected benefits. He is highly unlikely to think that his own future consumption must be subtracted to calculate the benefits. Many collective decisions might be listed concerning the allocation of resources to health in the same way. Who will be the beneficiary of these additional services is not known. Each person, therefore, will tend to evaluate the potential benefits in much the same way that he would a decision concerning his own expenditures for health; i.e., he will see no reason for deducting consumption, since he may be the one who will benefit from the expenditure. *Ex post* he may reason that saving someone else's life did not do him any good, but in advance of the event and in the absence of knowledge concerning who the beneficiary will be, the full value of the discounted earnings seems the appropriate basis for valuation.

Better health can increase the number of potential man-hours for production by reducing morbidity and disability, as well as by reducing

TABLE 1-4

Saving in Lives and Economic Value Accruing from
(a) the Actual Reduction in Death Rate of U.S. Males from 1929 to 1960 and
(b) a Hypothetical Reduction of the 1960 U.S. Rate to the Level of Sweden

| Age | U.S. Male Population 1960 (Thous.) | Death Rate* (per Thousand) | | | Number of U.S. Deaths (Thous.) | | | Lives Saved (Thous.) | | Economic Value of Lives Saved (Millions of $) | |
		U.S. 1929	U.S. 1960	Sweden 1960	at U.S. Rate 1929 (1)	1960 (2)	at Swedish Rate 1960 (3)	Actual Col.1-Col.2 (a)	Hypothetical Col.2-Col.3 (b)	Based on (a)	Based on (b)
Under 1	2,090	79.8	30.1	19.1	166.8	62.9	39.9	103.9	23.6	1,525	347
1–4	8,240	6.5	1.2	1.0	53.6	9.9	7.8	43.7	2.1	834	39
5–14	18,029	2.0	0.6	0.5	36.1	10.8	9.0	25.3	1.8	743	53
15–24	11,906	3.7	1.5	1.0	44.1	17.9	11.9	26.2	5.9	1,381	314
25–34	11,179	5.1	1.9	1.2	57.0	21.2	13.4	35.8	7.8	2,524	552
35–44	11,755	7.8	3.7	2.0	91.7	43.5	23.5	48.2	19.9	3,247	1,346
45–54	10,093	13.9	9.7	5.1	140.3	97.9	51.5	42.4	46.4	2,222	2,433
55–64	7,537	26.7	22.7	14.1	201.2	171.1	106.3	30.1	65.6	899	1,958
65–74	5,116	57.6	48.3	38.2	294.7	247.1	195.4	47.6	51.2	447	481
75–84	2,025	126.8	99.6	98.2	256.8	201.7	198.9	55.1	4.5	136	11
85 and over	362	256.0	208.4	236.0	92.7	75.4	85.4	17.3	-9.3	0	0
Total	88,331	16.2	10.8	8.4	1,435.0	959.4	743.1	475.6	219.5	13,958	7,533

Sources: For U.S. death rates, 1929, see U.S. Bureau of the Census, *Historical Statistics of the United States*, series B123–154; for 1960, see U.S. Public Health Service, *Vital Statistics of the United States, 1960, 1961*, Table 1C. For data on U.S. population, see U.S. Bureau of the Census, *1960 Census of Population*, U.S. Summary, General Characteristics, PC(1) 1B, Tables 45 and 46. For Swedish death rates, see *Annual Epidemiological and Vital Statistics, 1959, 1960, and 1961*, Table 4.

* Three-year average centered on year indicated.

mortality. Some estimate of the potential gains to the economy from this source can be obtained from data collected periodically as part of the National Health Survey. In 1964, approximately 5.5 workdays per person were lost for health reasons by those currently employed [70]. Additional loss was contributed by those persons who would have been employed except for reasons of health.

Health and Productivity

Common sense suggests that better health should result in more production per man, as well as more men available for work. Unfortunately, very little research has been done to provide a basis for estimating the magnitude of this effect. Company-sponsored health programs would seem to offer an excellent opportunity for the study of this question, but not much has been done. In one investigation of what executives *thought* were the results of their company's health program, "less absenteeism" was mentioned by 55 per cent of the respondents, "improved employee health" was mentioned by 50 per cent, but "improved productivity on the job" was mentioned by only 12 per cent of the respondents [47].

A number of studies have examined company health programs [10, 14, 20, 46], but their emphasis is on turnover rates, accident rates, absenteeism, and Workmen's Compensation insurance premiums rather than on output per man-hour. Whether this is because the latter effect is small or because it is difficult to measure is not clear. Many of the studies suffer from failure to consider other relevant variables along with the presence or absence of a company health program. Also, these studies do not clarify whether the benefits of company health programs should be attributed to improvements in health. For example, absenteeism and medical expenses may be lowered because of better controls rather than because of any change in health.

One special aspect of company health programs is the periodic health examination, much favored by those interested in preventive medicine. The basic notion is that if diseases or other injurious conditions are discovered early enough the chances for arrest or cure are greatly enhanced. An extensive literature exists on this subject, reviewed by Roberts [50], but, unfortunately, the studies do not clearly establish the economic value of such examinations. Roberts lists several values served by such examinations, but concludes that both public health service activities and personal health practices have much more effect on health than do periodic examinations.

A thorough economic analysis of the costs and benefits of company health programs and periodic health examinations is needed. Such an analysis should pay special attention to all the real costs of these programs, including, for example, the time demanded of the examinees. It should also attempt to distinguish between those benefits which are realized through improvements in health and those which are unrelated to health.

Health and Consumption

In contrast to the substantial number of studies that look at the economic value of health in terms of production, very little information is available concerning its value as an end in itself (consumption). Klarman has suggested that one way of approaching the problem would be to observe the expenditures that people are willing to incur for the elimination of nondisabling diseases or the expenditure incurred by those not in the labor force [26, p. 64].

Many people in the public health field greatly overestimate the value that the consumer places on health. The health literature frequently seems to read as if no price were too great to pay for good health, but the behavior of consumers indicates that they are often unwilling to pay even a small price. For example, surveys have shown that many people do not brush their teeth regularly, even when they believe that brushing would significantly reduce tooth decay and gum trouble [22, 25]. Smokers who acknowledge the harmful effects of smoking refuse to stop [60], and a group of executives whose obesity was called to their attention by their physicians took no action to correct a condition which is acknowledged to be injurious to health [77]. Some cases (mostly communicable diseases) may be noted where the social consumption value of health is greater than the private consumption value because of important external effects. The examples cited, however, do not fall into this category.

One of the problems that should be squarely faced in framing a social policy for health services is that people differ in the relative value that they place on health, just as they differ in the relative value that they place on other goods and services. Any system which attempts to force all people to buy the same amount of health services is likely to result in a significant misallocation of resources.

Health and Life Attitudes

This is another area where one can do little more than say that research would be desirable. Many people have speculated about the effect of changes in health levels on attitudes toward work, saving, birth control, and other aspects of behavior, but not much evidence has been accumulated. One interesting question concerns the ability of various populations to perceive changes in health levels. A study of low-income Negroes in Chicago revealed very little awareness that a significant decline in infant mortality had actually occurred [11]. This suggests that changes in life attitudes, if they are related to changes in health levels, probably occur only after a lag.

CONCLUSION

The principal line of argument in this paper may be stated briefly: health services represent the combined inputs of labor, capital, and intermediate goods and services used by the health industry. Their contribution to the economy must be measured by the output of this industry, which takes three forms: health, validation services, and other consumer services. Of the three, health is probably the most important. The problem of measuring changes in health levels is examined and the relationship between health services and health is discussed. Measuring the latter is greatly complicated by the fact that health depends upon environmental factors as well as health services. Most of the studies treat rising income as favorable to health, but some reasons are presented for questioning the validity of this assumption for the United States at present. The economic importance of changes in health levels flows, first, from the importance of health as a consumption goal in itself and, second, from the effect of health on production. This effect can take two forms—changes in potential man-hours and changes in output per man-hour. Changes in life attitudes attributable to changes in health levels also may indirectly affect the economy.

Throughout the paper the need for additional research on each of these concepts and relationships has been stressed. Many of the studies cited have also dealt at length with the question of needed research. The best stimulus to good research is a good example; exhortation is a poor substitute. Nevertheless, this paper will conclude with a few comments on possible points of departure for research.

One promising line of inquiry would be to capitalize on the fact that health services in this country and abroad are produced and financed under a bewildering array of institutional arrangements. Important differences may be found with respect to the ownership and control of facilities, the organization of medical practice, the pricing of health services, the remuneration of health personnel, and many other aspects of industrial organization. A basic question to be asked in each case is, "What are the implications of these differences for health and for the economy?"

Another potentially fruitful area of work concerns the advances in medical technology which are the principal source of productivity gain for this industry. The American Medical Association has compiled a list of "significant advances and technological developments" for the period 1936–62, by specialty, based on the response of knowledgeable physicians to a mail survey [4, vol. 3, pp. 4–12]. The same source presents a list of thirty important therapeutic agents now in use that have been introduced since 1934 [4, vol. 3, pp. 3–14]. Both could provide a useful departure for research on the costs and benefits of medical research as well as for studies of innovation and diffusion similar to those that Mansfield [36] and Griliches [21] have developed for other parts of the economy.

The introduction to this paper argued that one of the principal reasons for wanting to know something about the contribution of health services to the economy is to be able to make better decisions concerning the allocation of resources to health. These decisions are increasingly made by government and are implemented in the form of subsidies for hospital construction, medical education, and even medical care. This suggests that one line of fruitful research might be developed as follows:

1. The question of health versus other goals must be considered. Although lip service is often paid to the notion that health is a goal to be desired above all else, the most casual inspection of human behavior provides ample refutation of this proposition. Viewed as a source of consumer satisfaction, good health is often shunted aside in favor of the pleasure to be derived from objects of expenditure and other patterns of behavior. Although the path to better health is frequently portrayed in terms of more hospitals, more doctors, and more drugs, most people have the potential of improving their own health by their own actions. Ignorance may be cited to explain the failure of people to take these actions, but this is manifestly untrue in many cases (e.g., doctors continue to smoke). Furthermore, "ignorance" frequently means nothing more than that people have not taken the time or trouble to obtain readily available information about health.

Health also contributes to the economy through production, but alternative ways of increasing output are available. To cite two important ones, resources allocated to increasing health could be allocated to increasing the stock of physical capital, or to increasing the rate of technological change through research and development. Anyone arguing for greater investment in health to increase production should be prepared to show that the return to investment in health is greater than the return to alternative forms of investment.

2. Once a decision has been made regarding the allocation of resources for health relative to other consumer goals and alternative forms of investment, a second allocation decision is required to divide resources among health services and alternative routes to better health. For instance, expectant mothers may benefit from frequent visits to a board-certified obstetrician, but they may also benefit from a better diet, or from not having to work during the last months of pregnancy, or from having someone to help them with their other children.

One can think of health problems where the environmental factors are of negligible importance and health services can make the difference between life and death. However, many situations also exist where both the environment and health services have a role to play and, given a fixed amount of resources to be used for health purposes, knowing the relative contributions (at the margin) of each is important for an efficient allocation of resources.

3. The third and most detailed level of decision making concerns the allocation of resources among various types of health services. More doctors, more nurses, more hospitals, more dentists—in short, more of everything—is needed. Given the decision about resources available for health and the allocation of these resources among health services and other health factors, however, one must have some notion about the contribution (again at the margin) of various types of health services. The absence of such knowledge probably means that public decisions concerning increases of these services can be made only on an arbitrary basis. The argument that the various health resources must be increased in fixed proportion is refuted by the evidence from other countries where health systems are successfully using doctors, nurses, hospital facilities, and other health inputs in proportions that differ strikingly from country to country as well as from those used in the United States.

One final note of caution seems to be in order. Whatever research approach is pursued, and whatever questions are attacked, economists must become familiar with health institutions and technology. The practice of medicine is still more an art than a science. The intimate nature of the relationship between patient and doctor, the vital character of the service rendered, and the heavy responsibilities assumed by medical personnel suggest the dangers inherent in reducing health care to matters of balance sheets, or supply and demand curves. Economics has something to contribute to health problems, but it should proceed as the servant of health, not its master.

REFERENCES

[1] Altendorfer, Marion E. "Relationship Between Per Capita Income and Mortality in the Cities of 100,000 or More Population." *Public Health Report* 62 (1947): 1681–91.

[2] American Heart Association. "Treatment of Acute Rheumatic Fever in Children: A Cooperative Clinical Trial of ACTH, Cortisone, and Aspirin." *British Medical Journal* 1 (1955): 555–74.

[3] American Hospital Association. *Hospitals* 38, Guide Issue, Part 2 (1964).

[4] American Medical Association. *Commission on The Cost of Medical Care Report,* 3 vols. Chicago: The American Medical Association, 1963–64.

[5] "An Interview with J. Douglas Colman." *Hospitals* 39 (1965): 45–49.

[6] Andersen, Ronald, and Anderson, Odin W. "Trends in Personal Health Spending." *Progress in Health Services* 14, November–December 1965.

[7] Anderson, Alice L., and Altman, Isidore. *Methodology in Evaluating the Quality of Medical Care, An Annotated Selected Bibliography, 1955–61.* Pittsburgh: University of Pittsburgh Press, 1962.

[8] Arrow, Kenneth J. "Uncertainty and the Welfare Economics of Medical Care." *American Economic Review* 53 (1963): 941–73.

[9] Becker, Gary S. "A Theory of the Allocation of Time." *The Economic Journal* 75 (1965): 493–517.

[10] Blankenship, Marilyn. "Influenza Immunization and Industrial Absenteeism—A Seven-Month Study." *Proceedings of the Fourteenth International Congress on Occupational Health,* Vol. 2, pp. 294–95. Madrid: 1963.

[11] Bogue, Donald J. "Inventory, Explanation, and Evaluation by Interview of Family Planning: Motives—Attitudes—Knowledge—Behavior—Fertility Measurement." Document prepared for International Conference on Family Planning Programs, Geneva, August 23–27, 1965. Mimeographed.

[12] Brest, Albert N. "Treatment of Coronary Occlusive Disease: Critical Review." *Diseases of the Chest* 45 (1964): 40–45.

[13] Cain, Harvey D., et al. "Current Therapy of Cardiovascular Disease." *Geriatrics* 18 (1963): 507–18.

[14] Cipolla, J. A. "The Occupational Health Experiences of Two American Hotels for 1955 and 1956." *Proceedings of the Fourteenth International Congress on Occupational Health,* Vol. 2, pp. 290–91. Madrid: 1963.

[15] Combined Staff Clinic. "Recent Advances in Hypertension." *American Journal of Medicine* 39 (1965): 634–38.

[16] Denison, Edward F. "Study of European Economic Growth." Washington: The Brookings Institution. Mimeographed.

[17] Dunn, John E., Jr. "Cancer of the Cervix—End Results Report." *Fifth National Cancer Conference Proceedings,* pp. 253–57. Philadelphia: J. B. Lippincott Co., 1965.

[18] Farmer, A. W., and Shandling, B. S. "Review of Burn Admissions, 1956–1960—The Hospital for Sick Children, Toronto." *Journal of Trauma* 3 (1963): 425–32.

[19] Forshall, Isabella, and Rickham, P. P. "Experience of a Neonatal Surgical Unit—The First Six Years." *The Lancet* 2 (1960): 751–54.

[20] Grant, Ellsworth S. "The U.S. Concept of and Experience in Small-Plant Health Services." *Proceedings of Thirteenth International Congress on Occupational Health,* pp. 118–20. New York: 1960.

[21] Griliches, Zvi. "Hybrid Corn: An Exploration in the Economics of Technological Change." *Econometrica* 25 (1957): 501–22.

[22] Haefner, Don P., et al. "Preventive Actions Concerning Dental Disease, Tuberculosis, and Cancer." Paper delivered at the Twenty-second Annual Meeting of the Association of Teachers of Preventive Medicine, Chicago, October 17, 1965. Mimeographed.

[23] Johnson, R. H. "The Health of Israel." *The Lancet* 2 (1965): 842–45.

[24] Kaiser, R. F., et al. "Uterine Cytology." *Public Health Report* 75 (1960): 423–27.

[25] Kirscht, John P. "A National Study of Health Beliefs." Ann Arbor: University of Michigan, 1965. Manuscript.

[26] Klarman, Herbert E. *The Economics of Health.* New York: Columbia University Press, 1965.

[27] Krementz, Edward T. "End Results in Skin Cancer." *Fourth National Cancer Conference Proceedings,* pp. 629–37. Philadelphia: J. B. Lippincott Co., 1961.

[28] Kutner, Ann G. "Current Status of Steroid Therapy in Rheumatic Fever." *American Heart Journal* 70 (1965): 147–49.

[29] Lerner, Monroe, and Anderson, Odin W. *Health Progress in the United States 1900–1960: A Report of the Health Information Foundation,* p. 43. Chicago: University of Chicago Press, 1963.

[30] Lewison, Edwin F. "An Appraisal of Long-Term Results in Surgical Treatment of Breast Cancer." *Journal of the American Medical Association* 186 (1963): 975–78.

[31] Lindsay, Malcolm I., Jr., and Spiekerman, Ralph E. "Re-evaluation of Therapy of Acute Myocardial Infarction." *American Heart Journal* 67 (1964): 559–64.

[32] Lockwood, Howard J., et al. "Effects of Intensive Care on the Mortality Rate of Patients with Myocardial Infarctions." *Public Health Report* 78 (1963): 655–61.

[33] Long, A. P. "Immunization to Tetanus." *Recent Advances in Medicine and Surgery,* pp. 311–13. Washington: Walter Reed Army Institute of Research, 1955.

[34] Long, A. P. and Sartwell, P. E. "Tetanus in the U.S. Army in World War II." *Bulletin of the U.S. Army Medical Department* 7 (1947): 371–85.

[35] Lowenthal, Milton, et al. "An Analysis of the Rehabilitation Needs and Prognosis of 232 Cases of Cerebral Vascular Accident." *Archives of Physical Medicine* 40 (1959): 183–86.

[36] Mansfield, Edwin. "The Diffusion of Technological Change." *National Science Foundation Reviews of Data Research and Development,* October 1961.

[37] Marks, Herbert H. "Longevity and Mortality of Diabetics." *American Journal of Public Health* 55 (1965): 416–23.

[38] May, Philip R. A. and Tuma, A. Hussain. "Schizophrenia—An Experimental Study of Five Treatment Methods." *British Journal of Psychiatry* 111 (1965): 503–10.

[39] McKinnon, N. E. "The Effects of Control Programs on Cancer Mortality." *Canadian Medical Association Journal* 82 (1960): 1308–12.

[40] Meadows, Susan H. "Social Class Migration and Chronic Bronchitis: A Study of Male Hospital Patients in the London Area." *British Journal of Preventive and Social Medicine* 15 (1961): 171–75.

[41] Merriam, Ida C. "Social and Welfare Expenditures, 1963–64." *Social Security Bulletin* 27 (1964): 3–14.

[42] Morris, J. N. *Uses of Epidemiology.* 2d. ed., p. 14. Baltimore: The Williams & Wilkins Co., 1964.

[43] Morrison, S. L. and Goldberg, E. M. "Schizophrenia and Social Class." *Journal of Mental Science* 109 (1963): 785–802.

[44] Mushkin, Selma J. "Health as an Investment." *Journal of Political Economy,* supplement, 70 (1962): 129–57.

[45] ———. "Why Health Economics?" *The Economics of Health and Medical Care,* pp. 3–13. Ann Arbor: The University of Michigan Press, 1964.

[46] National Health Forum. "Are Occupational Health Programs Worthwhile?" In *Health of People Who Work,* Albert Q. Maisel, ed., pp. 11–28. New York: National Health Council, 1960.

[47] National Industrial Conference Board. *Company Medical and Health Programs,* Studies in Personnel Policy 171, p. 13. New York: National Industrial Conference Board, 1959.

[48] Reed, Louis S. and Rice, Dorothy P. "National Health Expenditures: Object of Expenditures and Source of Funds, 1962." *Social Security Bulletin* 27 (1964): 11–21.

[49] Roberts, Ffrangcon. *The Cost of Health.* London: Turnstile Press, 1952.

[50] Roberts, Norman J. "The Values and Limitations of Periodic Health Examinations." *Journal of Chronic Diseases* 9 (1959): 95–116.

[51] Rosen, George. "The Bacteriological Immunologic and Chemotherapeutic Period 1875–1950." *Bulletin of the New York Academy of Medicine* 40 (1964): 483–94.

[52] Sanders, B. S. "Measuring Community Health Levels." *American Journal of Public Health* 54 (1964): 1063–70.

[53] Schlesinger, E. R. "Dietary Fluoride and Caries Prevention." *American Journal of Public Health* 55 (1965): 1123–29.

[54] Schwartz, Samuel, and Vinyard, John H. "Prenatal Care and Prematurity." *Public Health Report* 80 (1965): 237–48.

[55] Shapiro, Sam, et al. "Comparisons of Prematurity and Prenatal Mortality in a General Population and in a Population of a Prepaid Group Practice." *American Journal of Public Health* 48 (1958): 170–87.

[56] ———. "Further Observations on Prematurity and Prenatal Mortality in a General Population and in the Population of a Prepaid Group Practice Medical Plan." *American Journal of Health* 50 (1960): 1304–17.

[57] Stout, John, et al. "Status of Congenital Heart Disease Patients Ten to Fifteen Years After Surgery." *Public Health Reports* 79 (1964): 377–82.

[58] Sullivan, D. F. "Conceptual Problems in Developing an Index of Health." *Vital and Health Statistics,* Public Health Service Publication 1,000, Series 2, No. 17. Washington: May 1966.

[59] Sutherland, Robert. *Cancer: The Significance of Delay,* pp. 196–202. London: Butterworth and Co., Ltd., 1960.

[60] Swinehart, James W., and Kirscht, John P. "Smoking: A Panel Study of Beliefs and Behavior Following the PHS Report." Paper delivered at the Annual Meeting of the American Psychological Association, Chicago, 1965. Mimeographed.

[61] Terris, Milton. "The Relevance of Medical Care to the Public Health." Paper delivered before American Public Health Association, November 13, 1963. Mimeographed.

[62] U.S. Bureau of Labor Statistics. *Study of Consumer Expenditures, Incomes and Savings, Volume VIII, Summary of Family Expenditures for Medical Care and Personal Care.* Philadelphia: University of Pennsylvania Press, 1956.

[63] ———. *Study of Consumer Expenditures, Incomes and Savings, Volume XVIII, Summary of Family Income, Expenditures and Savings, All Urban Areas Combined.* Philadelphia: University of Pennsylvania Press, 1957.

[64] U.S. Department of Commerce, Bureau of the Census. *U.S. Census of Manufactures.* Washington: 1963.

[65] ———. *U.S. Census of Population.* Washington, decennial.

[66] ———. *U.S. Censuses of Population and Housing: 1960, 1 / 1000, 1 / 10,000: Two National Samples of the Population of the United States.* Washington.

[67] U.S. Department of Commerce, Office of Business Economics. *National Income, 1954 Edition, A Supplement to the Survey of Current Business.* Washington: 1954.

[68] ———. *Survey of Current Business.* Washington, annual July issues.

[69] ———. *U.S. Income and Output, A Supplement to the Survey of Current Business.* Washington: 1958.

[70] U.S. Department of Health, Education, and Welfare, Public Health Service. "Disability Days: United States, July 1963–June 1964." *Vital and Health Statistics,* Series 10, No. 24, p. 16. Washington: 1965.

[71] ———. "Measurement of Personal Health Expenditures." *Vital and Health Statistics,* Series 2, No. 2. Washington: 1963.

[72] ———. "Personal Health Expenses; Distribution of Persons by Amount and Type of Expense, United States, July–December 1962." *Vital and Health Statistics,* Series 10, No. 22. Washington: 1965.

[73] ———. *Coronary Care Units: Specialized Intensive Care Units for Acute Myocardial Infarction Patients.* Washington: October 1964.

[74] ———. *Health Manpower Source Book,* Sections 1–19. Washington: 1952–64.

[75] U.S. Treasury Department, Internal Revenue Service. *Statistics of Income, 1962: U.S. Business Tax Returns.* Washington: 1965.

[76] The University of Michigan Department of Economics. *The Economics of Health and Medical Care.* Ann Arbor: The University of Michigan Press, 1964.

[77] Wade, Leo, et al. "Are Periodic Health Examinations Worthwhile?" *Annals of Internal Medicine* 56 (1962): 81–93.

[78] Wilson, May G., et al. "The Decline of Rheumatic Fever—Recurrence Rates of Rheumatic Fever Among 782 Children for 21 Consecutive Calendar Years." *Journal of Chronic Diseases* 7 (1958): 183–97.

[79] Wolf, Bernard M. "The Economics of Medical Research and Medical Care—From the Point of View of Economic Growth." Washington: Public Health Service, Resource Analysis Branch, 1964. Manuscript.

[80] World Health Organization. "Constitution of the World Health Organization, Annex I." *The First Ten Years of the World Health Organization.* Geneva: 1958.

[81] ———. *Expert Committee on Water Fluoridation, First Report,* Technical Report Series 146. Geneva: 1958.

[82] Wylie, C. M. "Participation in a Multiple Screening Clinic with Five Year Follow-Up." *Public Health Reports* 76 (1961): 596–602.

[83] Yankauer, Alfred and Lawrence, Ruth A. "A Study of Periodic School Medical Examinations." *American Journal of Public Health* 45 (1955): 71–78.

2

The Basic Forces Influencing
Costs of Medical Care   *Victor R. Fuchs*

INTRODUCTION

Until quite recently, an economist was rarely to be found in the company of the nation's leading physicians, and on those few occasions, he was likely to be flat on his back with one or more of his vital organs exposed to public view. It is my intention here to provide exposure of a different sort. The question—The basic forces influencing costs of medical care—is one which almost every physician would be prepared to tackle. My aim is to indicate how an economist goes about answering it. Economics is, above all else, a way of looking at questions. In Lord Keynes's words, "The Theory of Economics does not furnish a body of settled conclusions immediately applicable to policy. It is a method rather than a doctrine, an apparatus of the mind, a technique of thinking, which helps its possessor to draw correct conclusions."

To be sure, even among economists there is not always just one way of looking at things. Winston Churchill used to complain that whenever he asked Britain's three leading economists a question, he received four different answers—two from John Maynard Keynes. Nevertheless, there is a common fund of concepts, a common core of analysis, that nearly all economists use.

The basic analytical approach is a consideration of the factors affecting the demand for medical care and those affecting the supply—demand and supply, the two magic words. Some of us, when visiting hospitals, have discovered that by putting on a white coat and talking

NOTE: This material was presented in an address at the National Conference on Medical Care Costs, Washington, D.C., June 27, 1967.

rudely to nurses it is easy to pass as a physician. To be mistaken for an economist is often even simpler. All one need do is nod gravely and say "demand and supply."

Definition of Terms

Demand for and supply of what? I shall assume that medical care refers to the services rendered by physicians, dentists, and other health professionals, plus all the goods and services consumed in connection with their work, or upon their direction. Thus, the costs of medical care include the costs of hospitals, drugs, and the like. This lumping of diverse health services is a concession to convention and to the limitations of time. Ideally one should apply the demand-supply analysis separately to hospitals, dentists, drugs, and so on because the forces that influence the cost of one type of health service are often different from those that influence another.

What is meant by costs? At least three possible meanings can be distinguished. It could mean price, or cost of production, or expenditures. When people speak of the rising costs of medical care, they frequently are referring to rising expenditures, and this is the way I shall use the term.

Expenditure Trends

We all know that these expenditures have been growing rapidly. In round numbers, expenditures for medical care have risen from under $4 billion in 1929 to over $40 billion in 1965 and probably close to $50 billion in 1967. Even as recently as twenty years ago, expenditures were only $10 billion. Of course, expenditures for most other goods and services have also risen; it is therefore more meaningful for some purposes to look at the share of total spending allocated to medical care. This, too, has risen, from under 4 per cent in 1929 to about 6 per cent in recent years. Nearly all of this relative increase has occurred since 1947.

Before examining the factors responsible for this trend, it is worth noting that there is nothing wrong a priori with changes in industry and sector shares of gross national product. Indeed, such changes seem to be a natural concomitant of economic growth. For instance, the relative importance of agriculture has declined precipitously in most western countries. During the last half of the nineteenth and the first half of the twentieth century there was a significant rise in the relative importance of manufacturing. Now we are witnessing in this country the growth of what I have described elsewhere as the "first service economy."[1] If agriculture's share of GNP falls from over 9 per cent to under 4 per cent, as it did in the United States between 1947 and 1965, some other industries must show increases. There is no magic in the 4 per cent figure for medical care; it is now 6 and it could be 8 or 10.

Reasons for Concern About Costs

Why then should there be a national conference on the costs of medical care? Let me suggest three reasons for concern.

First, questions arise concerning the contribution that these increased expenditures make to health. Although we spend much more per person for medical care than any other country, we do not enjoy the highest health levels. On the contrary, many European countries have age-specific death rates considerably below our own. The relatively high infant mortality rate in this country is disturbing, and difficult to explain. The disparity in death rates for middle-aged males is even more shocking, and has more serious economic implications. In the United States, of every hundred males who reach the age of forty-five, only ninety will reach fifty-five. In Sweden the comparable figure is ninety-five. During this critical decade when most men are at the peak of their earning power, the U.S. death rate is double the Swedish rate, and higher than that of almost every western nation. It certainly seems legitimate to ask why. This is not necessarily with a view to spending less for medical care—I doubt if anyone can foresee a decline—but with a view to developing more effective use of the resources that we are now devoting to health.

A second reason why we should be concerned about medical care costs is the peculiar structure of the medical care industry. Most industries in the United States consist of profit-seeking firms actively engaged in competition with one another. The fundamental rationale of the American economic system is that the hope of profit (and the fear of loss) under conditions of open competition are the best guarantees of efficiency, appropriate price and rate of output, and fair returns to the various factors of production. By contrast, the medical care industry is organized along radically different lines. Nonprofit operations are the rule in the hospital field; there are severe restrictions on entry and competition in medical practice; and advertising and patent control dominate the market for drugs. Thus, there is no a priori basis

---

[1] Victor R. Fuchs, *The Growing Importance of the Service Industries*, Occasional Paper 96, New York, NBER, 1965.

for believing that the prices and quantities of medical care approach those that would result from perfectly competitive market conditions.

A third reason is that a large and still increasing portion of the cost of medical care is paid by third parties. In particular, the taxpayer is being called upon to pick up a substantial share of the bill. Because payment for medical care is increasingly regarded as a collective responsibility, it is natural and appropriate that there should be collective expressions of concern, such as this conference reflects, about the quantity and quality of medical care, and about its price.

These quantities and prices are determined by demand and supply. Let us consider each side of the equation in turn.

DEMAND FOR MEDICAL CARE

Economists say that the demand for any good or service depends upon relative prices, income, and tastes.

Price

How does price affect expenditures? Perhaps the most firmly established proposition about the demand for medical care is that it is relatively inelastic with respect to price. If the price rises relative to other prices, the decline in the quantity demanded will be proportionately less than the increase in price. The result is an increase in medical care expenditures. If, other things remaining unchanged, price rises by 10 per cent and quantity demanded falls by only 5 per cent, expenditures will rise by approximately 5 per cent. Some studies suggest that the price elasticity of demand for medical care may be as low as 0.2, i.e., quantity demanded declines by only 2 per cent when price rises by 10 per cent. But present knowledge does not permit fixing a specific value beyond saying that the elasticity is surely below unity.

An aspect of the price of medical care that is not widely recognized is that it really has two components. One is the nominal price charged by the physician or hospital; the other is the value of the patient's time.[2] For instance, the nominal price of a visit to a physician might be ten dollars, but the trip to and from his office, the wait, and the actual examination will probably take an hour or more. This time might be worth more or less than ten dollars depending upon the alternatives available to the patient.

Once it is understood that the price of medical care includes both

[2] Gary S. Becker, "A Theory of the Allocation of Time," *Economic Journal*, 75, September 1965, pp. 493–517.

components, a number of interesting implications become apparent. Even if no sliding fee scale is used, the total price of medical care tends to vary with earning power. The price is lower for retired people and the unemployed than for those with jobs, generally lower for women than for men, and so on. Also, even when the nominal price is reduced to zero, as under prepayment plans or socialized medicine, the true price is not zero.

Income

One of the factors to be considered in any demand study is real per capita income. During the past twenty years this has risen by over 50 per cent, and there is no doubt that the demand for medical care increases with income. What is less clear is whether the demand for medical care is elastic or inelastic with respect to income, i.e., whether a given percentage increase in income leads to more, or less, than the same percentage increase in medical care expenditures, other things remaining the same. This question is only gradually yielding to attack as more and better data become available and analytical techniques are sharpened. Some recent studies suggest that the elasticity may be significantly below unity, and few investigators believe that it is greater than unity. At most, the demand for medical care seems to increase approximately in proportion to income. If this is true, we cannot attribute any of the increase in medical care's *share* of total expenditures to rising income.

Insurance

A special factor that complicates the analysis of the demand for medical care is the growth of insurance and prepayment plans. Once a person is covered by such a plan, the effective price to him of additional units of medical care depends only upon the value of his time. This may explain a large part of the increase in the quantity of medical care demanded, and may also help explain the apparent insensitivity of insured consumers to increases in the nominal price of medical care. It is worth noting that hospital care has shown the most rapid rate of increase in expenditures, and it is hospital care that has been most thoroughly covered by insurance and prepayment.

The curious behavior of dental expenditures also offers support for this hypothesis. All the available evidence suggests that at any point in time the demand for dental care is more elastic with respect to income than is the demand for physicians' services.[3] Nevertheless, dur-

[3] See Morris Silver's essay "An Economic Analysis of Variations in Medical Expenses and Work-Loss Rates" below.

ing these recent decades of sharply rising income, expenditures for dental care have increased less than have expenditures for physicians' services. One possible explanation is the very small role played by insurance and prepayment plans in the dental field. Expenditures for eyeglasses and appliances and for drugs, two other components of medical care that are typically paid for directly by the consumer, have also risen much less rapidly than have expenditures for hospitals or physicians.

This should not come as a surprise. The advocates of insurance and prepayment had something like this in mind. They wanted to remove any financial barriers to obtaining medical care. But it is a basic law of economics that if you lower the price, the quantity demanded will increase. A critic of the British National Health Service put the matter cogently, albeit a bit strongly, in a recent issue of *The Lancet*: "If taxi fares and meters were abolished, and a free National Taxi Service were financed by taxation, who would go by car, or bus, or walk . . . the shortage of taxis would be endemic, rationing by rushing would go to the physically strong, and be more arbitrary than price, and 'the taxi crisis' a subject of periodic public agitation and political debate."[4]

This does not mean that insurance and prepayment should be abandoned. But it does suggest a need to discover techniques—possibly coinsurance, deductibles, or experience rating—to check prices and expenditures without interfering with essential health services.

Tastes

All factors other than income or price that affect demand are put by economists in a catchall category called taste. In the case of medical care, this would include the factors that affect the health levels of the population and the attitudes toward seeking medical care at any given level of health. Taste for medical care, therefore, would be related to: (1) demographic variables, (2) education, (3) environment, (4) ways of living, and (5) the genetic stock of the population.

Research on these matters is only in its infancy, and there are few reliable findings to report. We know that an increase in the proportion of elderly people in the population tends to increase the demand for medical care, other things remaining the same. The effect of increased education is unclear. It probably leads to improved health levels, and thus less need for medical care, but may also lead to greater demand for medical care at any given level of health.

[4] Arthur Seldon, "National or Personal Health Service," *The Lancet,* 1, March 25, 1967, p. 675.

Most observers believe that recent environmental changes, particularly the increase in real income per capita, have contributed to better health status. I think that this inference is incorrect. Some tentative findings from my research suggest that the environmental and life-style changes of the past two decades have had either a neutral or negative impact on health for most of the population. One piece of evidence in support of this hypothesis is the stability of age-adjusted death rates in the United States in the face of large increases in medical care and improvements in medical science.[5]

All these questions, however, are in need of more study. The National Center for Health Statistics is now developing vast new bodies of relevant data. A combined assault on these data by health experts and social scientists could yield information of great importance in our continuing efforts to understand and improve the nation's health.

Accounting Illusion

In concluding this discussion of demand, it should be noted that part of the observed increase in medical care costs is an accounting illusion. It does not involve any increase in real costs—only money costs. It is the result of an increase in the proportion of medical care produced and sold in the market, and a decline in the proportion provided outside the market by family, friends, and neighbors. Only the former is included in the GNP. A generation ago, a considerable amount of bed care and associated services for the sick were provided for at home. Surely there is relatively less of this today.

Some of the reasons for this shift other than increases in income and insurance coverage, are: (1) urbanization, (2) the fragmentation of the family, and (3) the increased labor force participation of women. We do not know how much of the increase in observed medical care costs can be attributed to this shift, but it may be substantial. One corollary is that "home care" programs and other current plans to transfer costs back out of the hospital will reduce the money costs of medical care by more than they will reduce real costs.

SUPPLY OF MEDICAL CARE

I turn now to the supply of medical care. In studying the supply side of an industry there are three main elements to look at. The first is the supply of the factors of production—labor and capital—flowing into the industry. The second is changes in productivity, and the third is

[5] See the essay "The Production of Health, an Exploratory Study" below.

the degree of monopoly control, or other market imperfections that may influence the supply actually available to consumers.

Supply of Productive Factors

With respect to the supply of labor going to the health industry, the crucial question is whether the industry has to pay inordinately high wages in order to attract an increasing fraction of the total labor force. There is some evidence to suggest that the answer to this is "no." In technical terms, the supply of labor for the medical care industry is very elastic.[6] This is true, incidentally, of most other industries as well. Except in the extremely short run, the U.S. labor force is highly mobile and adaptable; studies of interindustry differences in earnings consistently refute the hypothesis that expanding industries must pay unusually high wages to bid away labor from other industries.

Between 1950 and 1960 medical care employment rose by 54 per cent, compared with only 14 per cent for total employment. Throughout the postwar period the annual rate of increase has been about 5 per cent for medical care employment, compared with a little over 1 per cent for the economy as a whole. Despite this rapid expansion, wages for medical care personnel seem to have been rising at about the same rate as in many other industries. This last point has not been thoroughly documented, but seems to be a reasonable inference from the data available.

An analysis of the supply of capital to the medical care industry is much more difficult to undertake because most capital is used in hospitals, and most hospitals are nonprofit. Thus, the flow of capital is not determined by the rate of profit (as it is in most industries), but by government decisions and by philanthropy. It is possible, however, to devise methods of financing and reimbursing hospitals that would make the flow of new investment more responsive to market-type mechanisms. The Soviet Union and other socialist nations have been attempting to do precisely this with substantial portions of their "nonprofit" economies.

Productivity

Changes in the supply of any good or service, in the sense of changes in the price-quantity relationships, depend primarily on changes in productivity. It is a commonplace to argue that productivity in medical care has advanced less rapidly than in the economy as a whole; but in

---

[6] It certainly would be in the absence of medical licensure and other restrictions on entry.

the absence of reliable measures of the output of medical care this must remain a matter of speculation.

The development of such measures is an extremely difficult task because of our ignorance concerning the precise contribution of medical care to health. In addition, output is not limited to improvements in health but takes other forms, including validation services and the "hotel" aspects of hospital care.[7]

There is some reason to believe that the available measures understate the true output of the medical care industry. A visit to a physician today is surely more productive than one twenty years ago, and this is even more true of a patient-day in a hospital. On the other hand, it is possible that many of the expensive procedures that are now part of "best practice" techniques are really not worth the money in the sense that their marginal contribution is small and the same amount of resources used in other ways would yield more utility to the consumer.

The common practice of reimbursing hospitals on the basis of their costs, as under Medicare and many other public and private programs, appears to be an open invitation to inefficiency. At best, the ability of hospital management to improve productivity is imperfect because of the independence of the attending staff. Under present arrangements, almost no one has any incentive to be concerned with the efficiency of the hospital as a whole.[8]

Physicians

The physician plays a key role in the supply of all medical care; his decisions and behavior affect almost everything else. Physician supply is now more specialized than formerly. This growth of specialization is often attributed to exogenously determined advances in medical science, but such an explanation ignores the role played by changes in demand. Two hundred years ago, Adam Smith observed that the division of labor is limited by the extent of the market. The relevant market for any one physician's services has grown tremendously because of the growth of income and population, the increased concen-

---

[7] See the preceding essay in this volume.

[8] With few exceptions, each hospital is independently "owned" and managed. In other industries an exceptionally able manager may gradually come to exercise supervision over an increasingly large pool of resources through the growth of his firm, through mergers, and through establishment of branch plants; this pattern is absent in the hospital field. Also, it is much easier for inefficient management to remain in charge for long periods of time.

tration in urban centers, and improvements in transportation. All these trends would lead to increased specialization, even if medical technology remained static. Moreover, given an increase in real income people want to buy more medical service for any given health condition. One way of buying more service would be to visit several different general practitioners, or to visit the same one several times. Alternatively, one can buy more medical service in each visit through the use of specialists. The specialist in medicine usually has more, not merely different, training than a general practitioner. The more valuable the patient's time, the greater will be the demand for "high powered" doctors. This demand-induced growth of specialization is thus a cause as well as a result of advances in medical science. Without a specialized practice, without the demand for specialized equipment and procedures, these advances would probably come more slowly.

Physicians have frequently been criticized because of their high earnings and their alleged desire to restrict their numbers. Such criticism, it seems to me, does not go to the heart of the matter. Most of the difference between the earnings of physicians and those of other occupations should not be attributed to their control over entry and competition, but to their long hours of work, the lengthy period of education required, and the absence of pensions, paid vacations, and other fringe benefits. Moreover, physicians' earnings account for less than 20 per cent of total health expenditures, and whatever the extent of their monopoly return, it could only be a small part of this fraction.

A more valid criticism, it seems to me, can be directed against physicians for their opposition to changes in the methods of producing and financing medical care. The medical profession, or at least a significant and articulate portion of it, seems to believe that there can be rapid and far-reaching technological change without disturbing the traditional organization of medical practice. This belief is irrational. One clear lesson from economic history is that technological innovation means organizational change.

One final aspect of physicians' market control is the extremely narrow range of options available for someone seeking personal medical care. One bit of evidence is the size distribution of earnings in the entire medical care industry which can only be described as unnatural. Nearly all American industries have a distribution which reflects a fairly smooth vertical hierarchy of personnel. There are usually large numbers performing routine functions, and relatively fewer persons at each successive stage of increased power and responsibility. Only in the medical care industry do we find almost a void in the middle of the distribution and a peak at the high end.[9]

Whether consumers would use less expensive medical care personnel, if available, would depend upon a number of factors—the institutional setting and supervision, the presence of a financial incentive, and so on. That it is technically possible for professionals with fewer than ten to twelve years of training beyond high school to render useful medical care has been repeatedly demonstrated in a variety of settings.

As some of my earlier remarks suggested, patients with high incomes and patients with acute conditions would undoubtedly continue to seek the highest possible level of training and experience. But the demand for something less might be large in cases of chronic illness, or in isolated communities, or among those with low incomes.

New Medical Techniques

One special feature of the supply of medical care is the appearance of radically new medical techniques and procedures. Normally, when economists speak of the supply of a commodity they assume that the quality of the commodity remains unchanged. This is almost never strictly true, even for such staples as coal or wheat, but frequently the change in quality comes gradually and can be objectively measured, and an increase in quality can be thought of as a decrease in price.

In the case of medical care, some of the new procedures (such as renal dialysis and open heart surgery) are so radically different from anything previously available that they cannot conveniently be analyzed in this manner. Part of the increased expenditure for medical care is undoubtedly attributable to the appearance of these new techniques for treating conditions that simply could not be treated before.

SUMMARY OF THE DEMAND-SUPPLY ANALYSIS

What conclusions emerge from this analysis of demand and supply? By now it should be clear that cost is the result of many forces, that rising costs are not necessarily bad (or necessarily good), and that economists have some interesting questions to ask, but are far from being able to supply all the answers. Many of the estimates have a large range of uncertainty, but sustained scientific investigation can reduce that range and increase understanding.

[9] See "The Distribution of Earnings in Health and Other Industries" by Fuchs, Rand, and Garrett below.

If we take as our analytical task the explanation of why medical care now accounts for 6 per cent of gross national product instead of the former 4 per cent, the following developments all seem to have played a role:

1. An increase in medical care prices vis-à-vis other prices facing a relatively inelastic demand. These price increases are probably related to the institutional rigidities that surround the organization and production of medical care.

2. The growth of insurance, prepayment, and other forms of third-party payment.

3. A shift from nonmarket to market production. If we measured all costs, the increase for medical care would not be as great as the GNP accounts indicate.

4. The introduction of radically new medical techniques and procedures to treat conditions that formerly could not be treated at all.

5. More tentatively, I have suggested that there may be greater need for medical care now to offset changes in the environment and in ways of living that are detrimental to health.

There is, admittedly, considerable question about the relative importance of these various factors, but the new emphasis being given to research on these problems should help us to make the quantitative estimates that are needed for planning and control.

3

Improving the Delivery of
Health Services
Victor R. Fuchs

As a fair warning to the reader, it must be stated at the outset that the many things that are good and right about our present health care system will not be discussed here. Instead, I shall concentrate on what can be done to make it better. The problem of improving the delivery of health services will be discussed from three aspects. First, there is the question of improvement measured purely in medical terms, that is, more effective health care. Second, there is the problem of achieving a more equitable distribution of health services. And finally, I shall consider the question of how to attain greater efficiency in the production of health services.

Improvement in the quality of medical care is something for which doctors and scientists are constantly striving, and one might think that there is not much that an economist can contribute to these efforts. This is essentially correct. Finding a better way to treat herniated discs, for instance, is primarily a technological task; and we must rely on those with training in the appropriate technology for a solution.

There are, however, two things that an economist can say about this question of better health services. The first is to point out that the best solution to a problem from a technological point of view is not always best from a social point of view. The reason is that the best technological solution may require the use of more resources than some alternative solution, and the allocation of scarce resources among competing goals is essentially an economic problem, not a technological one.

Most physicians tend to define optimum care without regard to cost.

NOTE: An earlier version of this paper appeared in *The Journal of Bone and Joint Surgery*, 51-A, March 1969, pp. 407–12. It was originally presented as an address to the Thirty-sixth Annual Meeting of the American Academy of Orthopaedic Surgeons, New York City, January 22, 1969.

This would be acceptable if resources were not scarce or if people had no goal other than better health. But resources are scarce, and people do have other goals, and therefore the optimum amount of care must be redefined. In plain language, the optimum requires allocating existing resources between medical care and other uses so that the last dollar's worth spent in each use brings the same amount of satisfaction or benefit to the consumer. Some practicing physicians have a good intuitive grasp of this principle, but others ignore it or fail to apply it with consistency to the broad problems of health care.

Recently I heard a well-trained, dedicated physician speak about new techniques for early detection of breast cancer through mass X-ray screening. The talk was most interesting and enlightening until the physician started to assert that the program was "worth doing." At that point his statements bordered on the irresponsible, because it was apparent that he did not have a set of rational criteria for deciding whether a program was "worth doing" or not. Questions concerning benefits and costs (both monetary and nonmonetary) and the like had been given only casual attention.

Coming closer to home, consider, for instance, the treatment of fracture of the forearm in children. An economist at the Palto Alto Medical Research Foundation found that the cost of such treatment rose very rapidly between 1951 and 1965, not so much because fees of individual physicians or charges of individual hospitals had increased, but because of changes in the way particular cases were handled.[1] In 1965, there was much greater use of orthopaedic surgeons and much greater use of hospitalization. That these changes represented better medical care can be accepted without a doubt. The real question is whether the improvements in outcome were sufficiently great to justify the additional costs. Maybe they were; I am certainly not saying that they were not. I am simply trying to indicate the kind of question that will be asked of physicians with increasing frequency in the future. And please note that the answer that the saving of a single life is worth any cost is unacceptable. The actions of society belie this assumption in a thousand ways every day. Moreover, the choice need not be between saving lives or not, but between alternative programs, that is, allocating scarce resources in order to save as many lives as possible.

A second point worth noting about better medical care is that it is not synonymous with more care. A substantial amount of evidence is accumulating that points to widespread overprescribing, overhospital-

[1] A. A. Scitovsky, "Changes in the Costs of Treatment of Selected Illnesses, 1951–65," *American Economic Review*, 57, 1967, pp. 1182–95.

izing, overtesting, and overuse of surgery. The economist notes with concern that frequently financial incentives seem to encourage rather than discourage practices that are harmful to health as well as wasteful of resources. For instance, the data on the disparate amounts of surgery performed on federal government employees, depending upon the type of health insurance plan that they are enrolled in, are rather alarming. According to the latest report, government employees and dependents covered by Blue Shield have four times as many tonsillectomies as those covered in group health plans. They have twice as many appendectomies, and twice as much female surgery, such as mastectomy and hysterectomy. It is possible, of course, to interpret the data as saying that those enrolled in group practice plans are being denied needed surgery, but in either case such disparities deserve more careful attention from the medical profession than they have thus far received. If current methods of financing and paying for medical care are a significant source of difficulty, physicians and economists can work together to devise new institutional arrangements that will be conducive to better care.

A second aspect of improving the delivery of health services is concerned with providing a more egalitarian distribution. The traditional system in this country was based on ability to pay, tempered by philanthropy, and the benevolence and judgment of physicians and hospital administrators. We are now experiencing strong pressures to change that system in the direction of distribution more in accordance with medical need. The country seems to be reaching a consensus that health services should be more evenly distributed than in the past.

This question, too, is only in part an economic one. Decisions concerning what is fair or just distribution of medical care (or anything else) must be based primarily on normative judgments rather than positive analysis. However, given society's objectives with regard to distribution, the economist can indicate how the pursuit of these objectives may conflict with other goals, and he can help in the search for efficient methods of implementing the objectives. For instance, given current social attitudes, it might be more efficient to develop a systematic approach to subsidizing medical care for the poor instead of depending on the discretion of physicians. How then to proceed?

Some reformers would create a national health service. They would finance medical care out of taxation and would make it freely available to all, presumably on a first-come, first-served basis, like the public parks. Such an approach runs several risks. First, it might have some seriously unfavorable effects on the quality of medical care. This service, unlike many items we buy, must be produced on a local basis. Furthermore, the "product" is highly personalized. These characteristics suggest that reliance upon remote control and supervision would be a mistake. Second, it might well result in fewer resources being allocated to medical care, because this field would have to compete with all the others for a share of the federal budget. Those persons who value medical care more highly than other goods and services would find it difficult to allocate their budgets in ways that seem best to them. Finally, the idea of a national health service takes the goal of more equal distribution and drives it to the ultimate extreme in ways that are likely to be harmful to both freedom and efficiency. We should recall Lord Acton's comment on the French Revolution: "The finest opportunity ever given to the world was thrown away because the passion for equality made vain the hope of freedom."

A very different approach would be the creation of special health programs for the poor. This has the advantage of recognizing the obvious truth that the great majority of people must pay for their medical care one way or another and that little is to be gained by pretending that if it is paid out of taxes the cost is being borne by someone else. A major disadvantage to this approach is the unfavorable aspects of a sharply delimited two-class medical system. It may well be with medical care as with education that separate systems are inherently unequal.

My preference is for a system which would subsidize the premiums of the poor for membership in plans and groups that also serve large numbers of the nonpoor. The latter's premiums would be paid by themselves or their employers. Under such a system the physician would know only that a person was a paid-up member and would not be concerned with the source of the payment. Membership in some plan or group that at least meets nationally established minimum levels would be compulsory for all, but there would be free choice of plan or group wherever practicable, including the right to buy more than the minimum level if desired. If these plans and groups were truly consumer-oriented, and if they negotiated at arm's length with the producers of medical care regarding price and quality, I think most of the objectives of greater equality could probably be served without sacrificing efficiency and freedom.[2]

While I am on this subject, may I add that statements by well-meaning social reformers about the provision of "highest quality care to all" are unrealistic and probably do more harm than good. If we

---

[2] See my "The Growing Demand for Medical Care" below.

can assume that the President of the United States gets the highest quality care, it should be clear that the provision of that level of care for everyone is currently impossible. Furthermore, even if we were much wealthier than we now are, it would require the diversion of resources away from the production of other things that people would rather have. It is also clear that no useful purpose would be served by providing the President with less care simply to meet some arbitrary goal of equality. I use the President as an extreme example, but the same point applies down the line. Every health system in the world contains elements of inequality based on position, political connections, family ties, or other factors. A system that provides a floor for everyone but a ceiling for none does not strike me as being less just and probably would be a good deal more rational.

The third aspect of improving the delivery of health services concerns producing them more efficiently. Whatever the state of the art of medicine at any given time, and whatever the equity of the distribution pattern, a case can always be made for increasing the efficiency of production. This would result in either more medical care for the same amount of resources or the use of fewer resources to produce the same amount of medical care.

The fundamental problem is to design a more rational system of delivery. Some of the principal areas requiring attention are hospitals, physicians' practices, and drugs.

The problem of hospital efficiency is threefold. First there is the matter of improving efficiency within individual hospitals. It is very important to provide hospital boards and managers with the proper incentives. Present methods of reimbursement, based largely on cost, do not do this, and other methods must be found. One approach worth considering is reimbursement based on the average cost of a group of hospitals with similar characteristics. Under such a system, inefficient hospitals would be under strong pressure to bring down their costs, while efficient hospitals would find themselves with extra funds which they could spend to improve the range and quality of services offered. This is an oversimplification, of course, and great care must be taken to maintain standards when applying such formulae.

Greater efficiency in hospitals also requires more rational organization of the hospital industry. The traditional pattern of fiercely guarded independence for each hospital frequently serves to raise the costs of all. Some remedies are being sought through areawide planning. Systems of hospitals under common management and control might also improve efficiency. No other American industry clings so tenaciously to the single-establishment pattern of organization in the face of dramatic improvements in transportation and communication.

A third and equally important road to greater efficiency for hospitals is through more judicious utilization. It is a sad commentary on the present system that it took a severe bed shortage for physicians to discover that early ambulation and early discharge are actually better for the patient in many cases. Have all the potential economies of this type been explored? The average length of stay for hernia surgery is now about seven days, but in the Shouldice Clinic in Toronto the average stay is two to three days. I am told that their mortality and recurrence rates compare favorably with those of any hospital in the United States.

This leads to the question of efficiency in the practice of medical care by physicians. This is not a simple subject, partly because, as one doctor recently put it, the physician "has taken over the roles of priest, medicine man, and grandparent combined."[3] Many people who visit doctors are, to quote the same article again, "troubled primarily by symptoms arising from their own anxieties, depressions, or guilt." But this raises the question of how well-designed the long years of medical training are to deal with this type of problem? Could not counselors with shorter but more appropriate training be more effective, thus freeing the physician for those tasks that require his special abilities? Of course, the diagnosis of neurosis is not simple and probably requires a highly skilled physician who can rule out other possibilities. It should be feasible, however, to separate the diagnostic and therapeutic tasks.

While there is great concern about the so-called doctor shortage, little mention is made of the considerable waste and excess capacity. The waste is evident in the time physicians spend at tasks that could be performed by someone with considerably shorter, more specialized training. The pediatrician providing well-baby care, the gynecologist attending normal deliveries, and the internist treating common colds might be examples of this phenomenon.

The excess capacity exists primarily in surgery. If you have any doubts about this, just perform for some surgical field the following calculation.[4] Take the annual number of procedures requiring a skilled surgeon, divide by the number of procedures that a skilled surgeon could perform if he were kept occupied, and compare the result with the actual number of surgical specialists available.

---

[3] M. J. Halberstam, "Who Says Solo Practice is Obsolete?" *Medical Economics,* December 23, 1968.

[4] H. C. Taylor, Jr., "Objectives and Principles in the Training of the Obstetrician-Gynecologist," *American Journal of Surgery,* 110, 1965, pp. 35–42.

For surgery as a whole, the figures look something like this: In 1966 about eleven million operations were performed in hospitals in the United States. (Normal deliveries are not included.) There were about 50,000 physicians with primary specialization in surgery (excluding interns, residents, and fellows). If all operations were performed by surgeons, and this certainly was not the case, the average work load would have been about 220 operations per surgeon per year. In New York State, the average would have been 170 operations per surgeon.

There are, to be sure, many qualifications to be entered along with these calculations. An important part of the surgeon's work is diagnosis and preoperative and postoperative care. The surgeon who, upon careful examination, recommends against surgery may often be doing more for health than the one who never leaves the operating room. Also, some operations require more than one surgeon and one resident, and some surgery is performed outside hospitals. But after all allowances are made, including time for teaching and time for attending meetings. it does seem possible that American surgeons as a group may be operating at only about one half of capacity.

Some excess capacity in surgery is probably desirable; but how much? And who is to decide? Organized medicine seems to be saying, let the market decide; but we do not now have a free market for surgical services and I have never met a physician who wanted a free market once he understood what the term implied.

A third area of inefficiency in our present health care system is in the production and distribution of drugs. Consider the manufacturer. According to the latest *Annual Survey of Manufactures* (1966), an average dollar's worth of shipments from drug factories breaks down as follows: 23 cents goes for cost of materials; 7 cents for wages of production workers; 10 cents for other payroll; and 60 cents is allocated to profits, interest, advertising, depreciation, and the like. In most industries this residual category accounts for 20 to 30 per cent of the sales dollar, and even in an industry such as toilet preparations, the fraction spent for materials and labor is higher and the residual is lower than in drugs.

The reasons for this huge margin are too numerous and complex to discuss in detail here. It should be noted that the principal components are the highest profit rate of all manufacturing industries plus large expenditures for research and promotion. Many people believe that the remedy for this situation is a barrage of legislation. Some changes in law may be necessary, but perhaps the physicians themselves could accomplish a great deal. If physicians, who are the source of all prescriptions, became more concerned with questions of drug efficacy and drug cost, dramatic savings would be possible.

It is a commonplace to say that we are moving into a new era for medical care in this country. The implications for the physician can be frightening, but they need not be. It is true that the structure and organization of medical care will no longer be determined primarily by the psychological and financial needs of physicians, but a rational system will not ignore these needs. The design of a rational system requires more than technological skill. Some physicians must acquire sophistication concerning the allocation of scarce resources to multiple goals. The principles involved are not difficult to master, and it seems to me that medical care and society will be better served if physicians play a prominent role in laying plans for the future.

In summary, improvements in the delivery of health services require making medical care more effective, producing it more efficiently, and distributing it more equitably. These are all difficult problems. The effort, wisdom, and dedication demanded of physicians is far greater than that required of most men. On the other hand, they are drawn from the top ranks of the youth of each generation; they receive longer and more expensive training than any other professional; and they lay claim to and are accorded more privileges. I sincerely hope that they will be equal to the tremendous tasks that lie ahead.

PART II

MEDICAL CARE—
DEMAND AND SUPPLY

4

The Growing Demand for
Medical Care
Victor R. Fuchs

Recent years have witnessed a sharp upsurge of interest in the economics of health. On the one hand, physicians, hospital administrators, public health officials, and other health experts are becoming increasingly aware of the need to carry out informed systematic analyses of the problems of organizing, financing, and distributing health services. On the other hand, economists are discovering the tremendous economic importance and challenge of health care and are beginning to apply to this field the analytical tools and concepts that have proved useful in a large variety of other situations. One such concept is that of demand, and this paper attempts to analyze the growing demand for medical care.

The application of economics to medical care is not a simple matter. It is desirable, therefore, to define terms before the analysis is begun. Demand, to the economists, is a technical term with a fairly precise meaning. When an economist talks about the demand for medical care, or any other good or service, he is talking about a willingness and ability to pay. This term should not be confused with "need" or "want" or "desire," although these words are frequently used interchangeably

NOTE: An earler version of this paper was presented to the Second National Congress on the Socio-Economics of Health Care, Palmer House, Chicago, Ill., March 22, 1968 and published by the *New England Journal of Medicine*, 279, July 25, 1968, pp. 190–95. It was reprinted by the National Bureau of Economic Research and distributed as a supplement to their Report 3, December 1968.

The opinions and assertions contained herein are those of the author and are not to be attributed to the Bureau.

I am indebted to Richard H. Kessler, M.D., for comments, to Elizabeth Rand for research assistance, and to Lorraine Lusardi for secretarial assistance.

This paper is supported in part by grants from the Commonwealth Fund and the United States Public Health Service (grant 1 PO1 CH 00374–01).

with "demand" by lay persons. The concept of the "need" for medical care seems to me to be imprecise, and of little value for analytical purposes. In practice, it can cover everything from a lifesaving emergency operation to the removal of blackheads. At any given time, there is a continuum of "needs" for medical care. Moreover, for any given condition, the perception of need is likely to vary from patient to patient and from physician to physician. This is not to say that wants and needs are unimportant. They have a major role in determining demand, along with other factors such as income and price.

The second important point about demand is that it usually cannot be measured directly. What we observe are data on utilization or expenditures. These are sometimes used as if they were measures of demand; they are not. They are the result of the interplay of demand and supply, and a full analysis requires consideration of both factors. It may be possible, however, to use expenditure data to make inferences about demand. In round numbers, expenditures for medical care, broadly defined to include physicians' services, hospitals, drugs, and the like, have been growing at an average annual rate of about 8.0 per cent over the past twenty years. I shall try to analyze this increase in terms of changes in price, population, income, and other factors. All the statistics used in the analysis are presented in Table 4-1.

According to the Bureau of Labor Statistics, the price of medical care has been rising at a rate of 3.7 per cent per annum over the same period. Whether or not this is an accurate measure of the trend in prices for medical care is a subject of considerable controversy. Numerous critics have suggested that the Bureau price index overstates the true price increase because of a failure to take into account improvements in the quality and effectiveness of a physician visit or a patient day in the hospital. It has been stated that a more accurate measure could be obtained by calculation of the change in the cost of treating a specific episode of illness.

A California economist, Anne A. Scitovsky,[1] has done precisely that for the five fairly common conditions treated at the Palo Alto Medical Clinic and the Palo Alto-Stanford Hospital. The period covered was 1951 to 1965. The five conditions were acute appendicitis, maternity care, otitis media in children, fracture of the forearm in children, and cancer of the breast. The findings are surprising. For all five conditions the cost of treatment increased *more* than the Bureau of Labor Statistics

[1] Scitovsky, "Changes in the Costs of Treatment of Selected Illnesses 1951–65," *American Economic Review*, December 1967.

TABLE 4-1

Factors Contributing to Growth of Expenditures for Medical Care, 1947–67

Factor	Average Annual Rates of Change (%)		
	1947–67	1947–57	1957–67
Medical care expenditures[a]	8.0	7.5	8.4
Accounted for by:			
Rise in price of medical care[b]	3.7	3.7	3.6
Growth of population[c]	1.6	1.8	1.5
Growth of real national income per capita[c]	2.3	2.0	2.5
Decline in quantity demanded because of rise in relative price of medical care[d]	−0.2	−0.2	−0.2
Unexplained residuum	0.6	0.2	1.0

[a] U.S. Dept. of Commerce, *The National Income and Product Accounts of the United States, 1929–65, Statistical Tables,* Washington, D.C., August 1966. 1967 figures estimated from R. S. Hanft, "National Health Expenditures, 1950–65," *Social Security Bulletin,* February 1967.

[b] U.S. Dept. of Labor, Bureau of Labor Statistics, *Consumer Price Indexes for Selected Items and Groups: Annual Averages 1935–58 and December 1965 to September 1967,* Washington, D.C., 1967.

[c] President's Commission, *Economic Report of the President,* Washington, D.C., February 1968.

[d] My estimate (see text).

price index of medical care, which rose by 57 per cent; the median increase in the cost of treatment was 87 per cent.

The principal explanations for the difference, according to the Scitovsky study, were, first, the failure of the price index to include, until recently, several medical services that have risen particularly rapidly in price; these comprise laboratory tests, x-ray studies, use of operating and delivery rooms, and anesthetists' services. A second consideration was the closing of the gap between the customary fee and the average fee. The price index of the Bureau of Labor Statistics is based on what physicians report is their "customary" fee. The average of fees actually charged by physicians is usually somewhat below the customary fee because charges above that level are rare but there may be circumstances when a physician will charge a particular patient less than the customary fee. These circumstances were more numerous and important in 1947 than in 1967. From an economic point of view, the average fee charged, not the customary fee, provides a more accurate index of the price of medical services. The third source of difference was changes in methods of treatment. For example, there was an increase in the number of tests and x-ray studies. There was also an increased use of specialists. A few changes in treatment slowed down the rise in costs (for example, the reduction in home visits in cases of otitis media), but, on balance, Scitovsky suspects that the effect was in the direction of rising costs over the period studied. Economists would not regard such changes as a true price increase, *provided* the new procedures and personnel were sufficiently more effective to justify the extra expense. This matter of changes in treatment will be discussed later.

The problem of measuring the true course of medical care prices cannot be settled by one limited study, but the Scitovsky results do raise questions about the popular belief that the medical care price index is necessarily biased upward. If it is assumed that the index provides a reasonably accurate guide to prices, expenditures for medical care in constant prices (that is, the real quantity of medical care) have been growing at a rate of 4.3 per cent per annum. This rate is obtained by subtraction of the change in price from the change in expenditures. What explains this increase? One of the most obvious factors is the size of the population; this has been growing at a rate of 1.6 per cent per annum. Thus, the real quantity of medical care per capita has been growing at a rate of 2.7 per cent per annum. Changes in the age distribution of the population could also affect the demand for medical care, but the changes that have occurred over the past twenty years have been neutral in this respect. An increase in the relative number of persons over sixty-five years of age, who are large users of medical care, has been offset by an increase in the relative size of the school-age population, most of whom are small users.

To explain the growth of per capita demand, we turn next to changes in income per capita. This is one of the most important determinants of the demand for any good or service. When real income increases, so does the demand for most goods and services. For some items the increase in demand is proportionately less than the increase in income; for others it is proportionately greater. We call the first group necessities, and the second luxuries.

Several investigators have attempted to measure the relation between income and the demand for medical care.[2] This is not an easy task.

[2] P. J. Feldstein, "Research on Demand for Health Services," in *Health Services Research 1*, D. Mainland, ed., New York, Milbank Memorial Fund, July 1966, pp. 128–65.

The available evidence, admittedly imperfect, suggests that changes in the demand for medical care may be roughly proportional to changes in income. In other words, whereas some aspects of medical care are clearly necessities, others more closely resemble luxuries; the average falls about in the middle.

Between 1947 and 1967 national income per capita in constant prices grew at an average annual rate of 2.3 per cent. Other things being equal, this should have raised per capita demand for medical care by about the same magnitude. However, other things have not been equal. The price indexes show that medical care has become more expensive in relation to other goods and services at a rate of 1.7 per cent per annum. This price effect would tend to reduce the demand for medical care by an amount determined by the responsiveness of demand to price change (the price elasticity of demand). Again, we do not have precise estimates, but most investigators believe that the elasticity is quite low—that is, rising prices for medical care do not have much effect on the quantity of medical care demanded. I judge that the price effect might have resulted in a decline in the quantity of medical care demanded of about 0.2 per cent per annum. The combined effect of changes in price and population and the growth of real national income per capita explains most of the 8.0 per cent per annum rise in medical care expenditures, but does leave an unexplained residuum of 0.6 per cent per annum.

It is interesting to apply the same analysis to the subperiods 1947–57 and 1957–67. For the first ten years, the changes in population, income, and prices explain nearly all the change in medical care expenditures. The unexplained residuum is on the order of 0.2 per cent per annum, which is well within the range of possible error in these estimates. For the past ten years, however, when medical expenditures per capita have been rising at a particularly rapid rate, a similar adjustment for changes in income and price leaves a residuum of 1.0 per cent per annum. Thus, it is the unexplained growth of demand in the most recent decade that requires principal attention.

In the search for an explanation, it should be recognized that a large part of the demand for medical care is determined by the physician. It is the physician who suggests hospitalization, the physician who prescribes drugs, the physician who orders tests and x-ray examinations, the physician who calls in a consultant, and the physician who says, "Come back in a few days and let me take another look at it." Thus, the physician, in addition to being a supplier of medical care, is also the consumer's chief advisor on how much medical care to purchase.

I do not stress this point to raise the vulgar argument about the relation between demand and physicians' income. There may be a few in the profession whose judgments are influenced primarily by financial considerations, but this is not the basic problem. Frankly, if physicians were the colluding profiteers that their worst critics accuse them of being, they would raise prices far above current levels and would make more money with less work.[3]

The problem, as I see it, is that the physician's approach to medical care and health is dominated by what may be called a "technologic imperative." In other words, medical tradition emphasizes giving the best care that is technically possible; the only legitimate and explicitly recognized constraint is the state of the art. And it is more than just tradition. Medical school training has the same emphasis as continuing education for physicians. All this sets medical care distinctly apart from most goods and services. Automobile makers do not, and are not expected to, produce the best car that engineering skills permit. They are expected to weigh potential improvement against potential cost. If they do not, they will soon be out of business. Moreover, the improvements must be those as perceived by the consumer—which may be very different from those perceived by the engineer. What is true of automobiles is true of housing, clothing, food, and every other commodity.

Even in education, a field often compared to medicine, the same balancing of costs against improvements in quality can be observed. Most people know that it is technically possible to provide their children with a better education than they are now getting. But they also know that this will require additional expenditures for facilities and personnel—expenditures that they are unwilling to undertake.

This weighing of costs against benefits can be found almost everywhere in the economy, but when we come to health, there is a deep-seated reluctance to do it. In practice, to be sure, the situation is not so extreme. First of all, if the new treatment of choice is less expensive than the one it replaces, no conflict arises. When the new procedure is more expensive than the old, it may not be used for a number of reasons. The physician may not know about the new technic or may not consider himself competent to use it; the necessary supporting facilities and personnel may not be available; the physician may take into account the economic circumstance of the patient; the patient may apply pressure to the physician to hold down cost; or the physician may ex-

[3] M. Reder, "Some Problems in Measurement of Productivity in the Medical Care Industry," in *Production and Productivity in the Service Industries*, V. R. Fuchs, ed., New York, NBER, 1969, pp. 32–35.

plain the choices to the patient, and ask him to make the decision. The last happens frequently in dentistry, for example, where there are usually several different ways of treating a condition, and these different ways vary in effectiveness, permanence, appearance, and cost. The dentist will frequently sit down and discuss the advantages and disadvantages of each aproach, and tell the patient the price. Dentists do not assume that they must always provide the best possible care.

The physician, however, is usually under considerable pressure to use the latest procedures and the most elaborate treatment. Keeping abreast of new developments is a difficult task in itself and leaves little time for attention to costs. The need to appear up-to-date and the fear of malpractice suits if things turn out badly add further fuel to the engine of medical inflation.

It is a fundamental proposition in economics that decisions involving the allocation of scarce resources to competing goals require a weighing of benefits against costs. However, there is little in the training or motivation of a physician to impel him to think in these terms. In this respect he is not different from any technologically oriented person, but almost nowhere else in the economy do technologists have as much control over demand. About the only exception that I can think of is the influence exerted by the military in time of total war.

The analogy is instructive. When a nation is fighting for its life, all other goals are subordinated to that of winning the war. The problem then becomes a technologic one, and technologic consideration should rule. The principal difference between a technologic problem and an economic one is that in the former there is only one goal, whereas the latter involves a multiplicity of goals.

If the American people were intent on extending life expectancy, or freedom from disease, or some other dimension of health to the maximum, they would seek the solution by bringing the best medical knowledge to bear on the problem and employing all necessary and available resources to that end. But the American people are clearly not intent on improving health to the exclusion of other goals. Thus, every time we urge that another billion dollars' worth of resources be used for health, it must be because the benefits from these expenditures are expected to be greater than those that would be realized if the resources were used for housing, education, or some other purpose. To the extent that medical care is involved in life or death situations, a similar dominance of technologic over economic consideration should prevail. But surely a substantial fraction of the $50 billion spent for health last year did not involve matters of life or death.

We must be careful not to underestimate the complexity of the problem under discussion. Tests, x-ray studies, and other procedures are frequently undertaken for their value in teaching, or for their possible contribution to medical knowledge, rather than in the expectation that they will provide immediate benefit to the particular patient. The ethical and legal questions raised in such cases are important but cannot be considered here. Of immediate concern is the question of how physicians can be brought to consider the economic as well as the medical consequences of their decisions.

Would such considerations inhibit the growth of new medical knowledge? Not necessarily. Much of the preference for the new, more complicated, more expensive procedures comes about not because medical knowledge has grown so much, but because it has grown so little. In many cases it is thought that one procedure is superior (in a purely technologic sense) to another, but what one would really like to know is *how much* superior it is in terms of *end results*. Good decision making in health, as in any field, requires the weighing of additional (economists call them marginal) benefits against the additional (marginal) costs. To implement this process in the medical care field, it will be necessary to acquire considerable medical knowledge of the differential in results obtained with alternative procedures.

The increased demand for medical care is only one aspect of a complex set of health problems. The medical profession is facing unprecedented challenges to raise the quality of medical care, to produce it more efficiently, and to distribute it more broadly. Unfortunately, much of the debate seems to take the form of refighting old battles. In economics the expression "bygones are bygones" is a short-hand way of remembering that the costs of yesterday are irrelevant to the decisions that must be made today. The only costs that matter are current and future ones. How rewarding it would be if that same attitude could be applied to efforts to devise a better system of health care! How refreshing it would be if physicians, government officials, economists, and other experts could move forward together in that spirit!

We are close to the beginning of a new day for medical care in the United States. If we can quiet our fears and restrain our passions, if we can credit the other fellow with a modicum of good sense and a sprinkling of good will, if we can forget the battles of the past and concentrate on the problems of today and the promises of tomorrow, we can be true both to ourselves and to our responsibilities to the American people.

5

Patient Characteristics, Hospital Characteristics, and Hospital Use

What would be the usefulness of the economics of consumption in a study of the consumption of services where consumer ignorance is large and the nature of the product poorly understood? What would be the influence on consumption of the usual choice-conditioning factors, such as demographic factors, socioeconomic factors, taste variables, and prices, in a supplier-dominated industry?[1] Would it be desirable or necessary to reverse the emphasis from demand to supply in order to investigate the consumption of such a product? This paper is an attempt to answer these questions by proposing a model and testing its usefulness with empirical evidence from the hospital industry.

In the hospital industry, consumers are pictured as making few or no choices because they depend entirely on the judgment of experts as to the desirability and the nature of the product they buy, and they cannot buy the product even if they are willing to pay for it unless

NOTE: This article appeared in *Medical Care,* 7, July–August 1969. It was originally presented at the 96th Annual Meeting of the American Public Health Association, Detroit, November 1968.

Research was conducted at the National Bureau of Economic Research, supported by grants from the Commonwealth Fund and the U.S. Public Health Service (Grant 1 PO1 CH 00374–01).

The author wishes to thank Victor R. Fuchs and Morris Silver for their valuable comments; Blue Cross of Western Pennsylvania for making the data available to him; and Susan Crayne for computer programing and other valuable assistance.

[1] On the choice-conditioning factors, see R. P. Mack, "Economics of Consumption," in B. F. Haley, ed., *A Survey of Contemporary Economics,* Homewood, Illinois, R. D. Irwin, Inc., 1952, pp. 49–63.

physicians authorize the purchase. The medical profession has promoted the idea that, given one's medical condition, the type and amount of hospital services provided are dictated by the "technological imperatives." Any variations in hospital use which are not explained by the differences in patients' medical conditions are attributed to the differences in the medical philosophies of the attending physicians and to "extramedical" factors such as age and sex of the patient.

Recent studies, however, have revealed two sets of systematic relationships—one between the patterns of hospital use and the socioeconomic characteristics of patients and the other between hospital use and hospital characteristics.[2] Partly in an attempt to explain the above relationships and partly as a separate theoretical development two distinct theories of economics of consumption of hospital services have emerged.

One theory postulates that hospital use is determined through the interaction between patients and doctors. A physician is described as treating a whole patient as a person, not a disease. Accordingly, personal and situational factors, in addition to medical conditions, are taken into consideration by doctors. These extramedical factors resemble the usual choice-conditioning factors listed in economics of consumption. The only departure from the traditional theory of con-

---

[2] There is a burgeoning literature on the relationship between hospital use and patient characteristics. Extensive references are provided in *Hospital Utilization Studies: Selected References Annotated,* U. S. Department of Health, Education and Welfare, 1962. U. S. Public Health Services also periodically publish the results of surveys on the subject through the National Center for Health Statistics Series. The most relevant issues are Series 13, numbers 1 to 3, and Series 10, numbers 20 and 30, *Vital and Health Statistics,* National Center for Health Statistics, U. S. Public Health Services, Department of Health, Education and Welfare. The other well-known surveys in the field are those by the Health Information Foundation—National Opinion Research Center; O. W. Anderson and J. J. Feldman, *Family Medical Costs and Voluntary Health Insurance: A Nationwide Survey,* New York, McGraw-Hill Book Company, 1956; O. W. Anderson, P. Colette, and J. J. Feldman, *Changes in Family Medical Care Expenditures and Voluntary Health Insurance: A Five-year Resurvey,* Cambridge, Harvard University Press, 1963; and R. Andersen and O. W. Anderson, *A Decade of Health Services,* Chicago, University of Chicago Press, 1967.

The relationship between hospital characteristics and hospital use has been studied in C. G. Skinner, "Hospitals and Allied Institutions," in W. J. McNerney, *Hospital and Medical Economics,* Chicago, Hospital Research and Education Trust, 1962, chapter 43; and D. C. Riedel, and T. B. Fitzpatrick, *Patterns of Patient Care,* Ann Arbor, University of Michigan, 1964, chapter 2.

sumer behavior is that it is the doctor who purchases the product on behalf of the consumer as an agent with "power of attorney" and that it is the responses of physicians to the choice-conditioning factors, not those of consumers themselves, that determine the consumption of hospital services.

The other theory is that economics of consumption has no role in explaining hospital use. Production of hospital services is envisioned as largely determined by technological imperatives and productive facilities available as well as institutional characteristics of individual hospitals. Consumers come into the picture only because their medical conditions dictate the product-mix of individual hospitals, but their wishes and expectations do not affect hospital use. The physician plays the pivotal role of the production manager who, using his knowledge of technology, combines factors of production to produce the "cure" of disease. In other words, given patients' medical conditions and technology, the physicians' responses to the environmental characteristics of individual hospitals determine the patterns of hospital use.

The model proposed is based on an integration of the two theories. Consumption of hospital services is hypothesized as a composite effect of the joint interaction among physicians, patients, and hospitals. The direct interaction is envisioned as taking place between physicians and patients. Hospital characteristics come into the picture as a factor influencing this interaction. The medical condition and socioeconomic background of a patient shape his expectations and wishes concerning hospital use. In the process of transmitting these, the patient reformulates them according to his attending physician's responses and the environmental characteristics of the hospital to which he is admitted. As for the doctor, his response is conditioned by his professional and personal background.

FORMULATION OF THE MODEL

Outline of the Model

In order to make the model operational, it is simplified and formalized as follows. The amount and type of hospital services provided are determined by the responses of physicians to the medical condition of patients, the socioeconomic characteristics of patients, the institutional environment of individual hospitals, and the interaction between patient characteristics and hospital characteristics. Four relationships constitute the basis of the model.

72

$$\bar{C} = \phi(M) \tag{1:0}$$

$$P = F_i(X_1 \ldots X_n),\ U \tag{2:0}$$

$$H = F_j(Y_1 \ldots Y_n),\ U \tag{3:0}$$

$$C - \bar{C} = \sum_i \frac{\partial C}{\partial X_i} X_i + \sum_j \frac{\partial C}{\partial Y_j} Y_j + \sum_{ij} \frac{\partial^2 C}{\partial X_i Y_j} X_i Y_j \tag{4:0}$$

where

$\bar{C}$ = the standard hospital use prescribed for illness M as "technologically" determined;

P = deviations from $\bar{C}$ caused by physicians' responses to patient characteristics;

H = deviations from $\bar{C}$ caused by physicians' responses to hospital characteristics;

X_i = patient characteristics;

Y_j = hospital characteristics;

C = total hospital use by patients with illness M;

F_i, F_j = behavioral relationships;

ϕ = a technology coefficient;

U = error term to make relationships stochastic.

The consumption of hospital services is measured by three indices: number of days hospitalized; weighted number of services received; and amount of the hospital bill. M, the medical condition, is represented by the final diagnosis recorded at the time of a patient's discharge from the hospital.

Patient characteristics are represented by six categories of variables:

X_1 = a vector of the demographic factors—age, sex, and race;

X_2 = income;

X_3 = method of payment;

X_4 = availability of substitutes for hospital care (as represented by proxy variables);

X_5 = cost of time spent hospitalized (as expressed by proxy variables);

X_6 = taste factors (as represented by proxy variables).

Hospital characteristics are also represented by six categories of variables:

Y_1 = peculiarities of individual hospitals (as expressed by dummy variables);

Y_2 = availability of hospital beds (as expressed by occupancy rate and the number of beds);

Y_3 = comprehensiveness of care provided (as expressed by weighted number of facilities and programs available);

Y_4 = availability of substitutes for inpatient care (as expressed by the existence or absence of an outpatient clinic and an organized home care program);

Y_5 = training activities of hospital (as expressed by the presence or absence of a graduate medical training program and a nursing school);

Y_6 = labor-capital ratio (as represented by proxy variables).

Some Problems in Applying the Data to the Model

In this model, the hospitals are depicted as producing the "cure" of diseases and illnesses using various factors of production operating under a given technology. (Training and research activities of hospitals are not discussed here.) It is assumed that, for each category of illness, there is a prescribed method of treatment, a method of producing the "cure." Thus, there is a production function for each "product," and the selection of a particular combination of factors of production, as expressed by the amount and type of hospital services provided, is determined by the physicians' responses to patient characteristics and hospital characteristics.

In measuring consumption of hospital care, therefore, a method had to be devised to measure, on a uniform scale, types and amounts of hospital services produced and simultaneously consumed. This necessitated formulating an output measure for the hospital industry. Hospital output is, however, an elusive concept difficult to define and measure.[3] Accordingly, although the proposed model takes the cure of disease as the conceptual unit of consumption, three input measures are taken as proxy variables for output.[4]

In a study of economics of consumption in the hospital industry, the use of input as the unit of consumption has this justification. Since consumers know little of the product they buy, they do not generate a demand for hospital care with a well-defined output, but instead in input terms, such as days of hospitalization, physicians' visits, specific procedures, etc. Furthermore, the three units of consumption adopted in this study—days of hospitalization, weighted number of services, and hospital bill—have traditionally enjoyed widespread acceptance,

[3] Of all the issues raised at a conference of experts, the problem of defining and measuring the product of the health industry was recorded to be most elusive and frustrating. See A. R. Somers and H. M. Somers, "A Program for Research in Health Economics," a paper prepared for a conference of experts, October 29, 1965, Brookings Institution, in U.S. Public Health Service Publication No. 947, Health Economics Series No. 7, January 1967, pp. 37–39.

[4] There are two positions regarding the output of a physician. Griliches argues that the doctor produces a "cure" and therefore a transaction unit should be the cure of a given disease. Gilbert, on the other hand, argues that the doctor produces an office visit, which should be the output measure. I take Griliches's position conceptually, but in measuring output, input variables are used. See Z. Griliches, "Notes on the Measurement of Price and Quality Changes," in *Models of Income Determinations,* Studies in Income and Wealth, Volume 28, Princeton, Princeton University Press for NBER, 1964, pp. 399–403; and M. Gilbert, "The Problem of Quality Changes and Index Numbers," *Monthly Labor Review,* September 1961, pp. 994–95.

and measure different aspects of consumption.[5] Thus, used together, they present a composite picture of hospital use.

Given each category of disease, ϕ in equation (1:0) purports to show the amount and type of hospital use technologically required to cure it. It cannot, however, be interpreted strictly as a technology co-efficient, for there is a broad area where individual judgment is exer-cised in producing the cure within each technologically prescribed method of treatment. This is what the medical profession calls the justifiable differences in medical philosophies of physicians.[6]

As a technology coefficient, ϕ also has a limited applicability be-cause of the problems of classification of "medical conditions." First, what constitutes medical conditions and what extramedical or personal situations is subject to interpretation. Second, how far the classification of diseases should be carried out poses a problem. On the one hand, a case can be made for treating every patient as having a different disease with a different medical requirement. In this case, ϕ as a technology coefficient loses its usual meaning because a new coefficient would have to be discovered for each new product. On the other hand, if classification is too broad, what appears to be the tolerance range in coefficients is in fact the difference in coefficients necessitated by producing different products.

In this study, for convenience and because of data restrictions, all cases are grouped into thirty categories of diseases following the In-ternational Code of Diseases Classification. Each category is further divided into four groups: surgical, nonsurgical, single diagnosis, and multiple diagnosis. Our technology coefficient, then, provides the standard (the mean value of) hospital use for one of the 120 groups thus classified.

In estimating the behavioral relationships behind F_i and F_j, the greatest handicap is the lack of information about physician charac-teristics. F_i purports to show physicians' responses to patient charac-teristics (X_i), and F_j, to hospital characteristics (Y_j). But even for

[5] Historically, these have been used as a basis to define and measure medical progress, as reflected in the changing pattern of hospital care and the cost be-havior of the hospital industry. For a comprehensive list of indices and measures of hospital use, see T. B. Fitzpatrick and D. C. Riedel, "Some General Com-ments on Methods of Studying Hospital Use," *Inquiry*, 1, 1964, p. 50.

[6] Once it is established that the understanding and practice of the "technological imperatives" do not necessarily lead to identical methods of treatment by indi-vidual physicians, what constitutes the quality of care is subject to individual judgment. See A. Donabedian, "Evaluating the Quality of Medical Care," Part 2, *Milbank Memorial Fund Quarterly*, 44, 1966, p. 166.

identical X_i and Y_j, it has been hypothesized that physicians' responses would vary. Since no data about physicians are available, hospital dummy variables are inserted instead. To the extent that physicians in the same hospital share common backgrounds and medical philosophies, hospital dummy variables would show the variations in physicians' responses attributable to variations in characteristics of physicians.

In equation (4:0), the interaction term $(X_i\, Y_j)$ is included because the model hypothesizes systematic relationships between some patient characteristics and some hospital characteristics. The problem of intercorrelation between the predictors is seen to exist because hospital characteristics influence the interaction between physicians and patients, and also because patients with certain socioeconomic backgrounds seek hospitals with certain characteristics by choosing doctors who have staff privileges in the hospitals to which they want to be admitted. Introducing the interaction terms is not expected to solve the complex three-way relationships hypothesized, in particular those due to lack of information about physicians' characteristics. The interaction terms are inserted in the hope that they may provide new insight into which variables interact and how.

Coverage

The subjects studied consisted of twenty-two hospitals in the Pittsburgh area and 9,000 patients admitted to these hospitals during 1963. The available data relating to the hospital characteristics include numbers of beds, occupancy rates, types of programs offered and facilities available, medical and nursing education programs, and financial data. Data relating to patient characteristics include demographic and socioeconomic variables and those from medical records (such as diagnoses), numbers and types of services received, numbers and types of operations, if any, amounts of hospital bills, sources of payment of the bills, types of insurance coverage, if any, et cetera.

The data were collected by Blue Cross of Western Pennsylvania. The principal method of analysis is the least-squares single regression in various forms and its variants, such as the two-stage estimation procedure.

RESULTS

Hospital Characteristics and Hospital Use

As expected, hospital characteristics more successfully explain the variations in hospital use when unadjusted measures are used than when the measures adjusted for diagnoses are used. This indicates a systematic relationship between the diagnosis-mix of an individual hospital and its characteristics as represented by these variables (see Table 5-1).

Differences in the characteristics of individual hospitals affect the patterns of special services provided and the hospital charges billed to patients more than does the length of stay of the patients. This is to be expected because the different medical philosophies of individual hospitals are more likely to be evident in patterns of care and price policy than in length of stay. This idea is supported by other regressions. Interhospital differences in hospital use are greatest when hospital use is measured by the weighted number of services, less when it is measured by hospital charges, and least when it is measured by length of stay.

Substitution of outpatient care and, to a lesser extent, (organized) home care for inpatient care takes place when these substitutes are available. Patients treated at hospitals which have outpatient clinics were hospitalized for shorter periods, received fewer services, and were charged less for inpatient care than those treated at hospitals without outpatient clinic facilities. This indicates that doctors who have staff privileges at hospitals which adhere to the concept of integrated care, providing intensive care, intermediate care, ambulatory care, and home care, do in fact substitute outpatient care for inpatient care at the diagnostic and convalescent stages of the patient's illness.

Patients admitted to hospitals which have graduate medical training programs receive significantly more hospital care—however measured— than those admitted to hospitals without such programs. For the most part, postgraduate medical training is carried out by larger hospitals with more comprehensive facilities. (The correlation coefficient between the number of beds and the weighted number of facilities is 0.66.) The greater use of hospital care by the patients in teaching hospitals may, therefore, be the result of these hospitals having more serious cases. To the extent that adjusting for differences in diagnoses failed to take into account the different medical requirements of patients, a positive relationship between the presence of the training programs and hospital use could be partly attributable to the differences in case-mix. A similar observation can be made about the significant positive relationship found between the weighted number of facilities of a hospital and hospital use by patients.

The presence of an accredited nursing school operated by the hospital appears to have different effects on hospital use from that of a

TABLE 5-1

Hospital Characteristics and Hospital Use, Adjusted for Differences in Diagnoses (n = 8986) Double Log

Hospital Characteristics	Length of Stay, Adjusted		Total Services, Adjusted		Total Bill, Adjusted	
	b Coefficient	Standard Error	b Coefficient	Standard Error	b Coefficient	Standard Error
Occupancy rate	-0.1507	0.0953	0.0421	0.0855	-0.0441	0.0838
Number of facilities, weighted	0.2969[b]	0.0549	0.4589[b]	0.0493	0.2358[b]	0.0483
Presence of intern program	0.1519[b]	0.0406	0.0493	0.0364	0.1068[b]	0.0357
Presence of residency program	0.1424[b]	0.0395	0.1362[b]	0.0355	0.2167[b]	0.0348
Presence of nursing school	-0.0485	0.0339	0.0913[b]	0.0305	-0.0804[b]	0.0399
Employees per bed	-0.2849[b]	0.0824	0.2284[b]	0.0740	-0.0175	0.0725
Presence of home-care program	-0.1375[b]	0.0224	-0.0534[b]	0.0201	0.0324	0.0197
Presence of outpatient clinic	-0.2462[b]	0.0561	-0.2668[b]	0.0503	-0.1874[b]	0.0493
a-constant	-1.1446		-1.7218		-1.1367	
Multiple R	0.11327		0.19356		0.12200	
R-SQ	0.01283[b]	(F = 14.6)	0.03747[b]	(F = 43.7)	0.01488[b]	(F = 17.0)
Adjusted R-SQ	0.01195	(DF = 8978)	0.03661	(DF = 8978)	0.01401	(DF = 8978)

[a] Significant at the 5 per cent level.
[b] Significant at the 1 per cent level.

graduate medical program. Whereas patients in hospitals with medical training programs stayed longer, received more special services, and paid more than those in hospitals without these programs, patients in hospitals with nursing schools stayed significantly shorter periods of time and were billed less, but received a greater number of services for given illnesses than those in hospitals without nursing schools. This may be because all the hospitals (nine of twenty-two in the sample) with nursing schools have residency and internship programs, but not vice versa. Just as hospitals with medical training programs are usually larger and more comprehensive than those lacking such programs, the hospitals with nursing schools are larger than those without them. (Hospitals with nursing schools had an average of 444 beds; those without one but with medical training programs, 190 beds; those without either, 178 beds. The mean weighted numbers of facilities of the above three types of hospitals were 45, 44, and 36, respectively.)

The distinctive patterns of patient care in larger hospitals with more comprehensive facilities seem to result in their patients receiving relatively more service-intensive and less time-consuming care. (The correlation coefficient between the weighted number of facilities and the number of special services, adjusted for diagnoses, is 0.102.) It appears that patients in hospitals with nursing schools are billed less for given episodes of illnesses because the savings realized from receiving daily hotel-type services for shorter stays are greater than the extra costs of the greater number of services received during the patient's stay.

Patients at hospitals with higher staffing ratios (employees per bed with occupancy held constant) are more likely to receive service-intensive care than time-consuming care. This conclusion is reached from the fact that patients at hospitals with high staffing ratios are hospitalized for significantly shorter periods of time for given illnesses than those at hospitals with low staffing ratios, but they receive greater numbers of special services.

The service-intensive care provided by hospitals with high staffing ratios was to be expected from the usual association between input mix and output mix. To the extent that the number of employees per bed represents the labor-capital ratio, the more employees per bed a hospital has, the more labor-intensive goods it is expected to produce. Since hospitals are a service industry, labor-intensive goods denote service-intensive care, that is, more things are done to each patient and less reliance is placed on the natural healing process.

To the extent that a higher staffing ratio is regarded as a desirable characteristic of a hospital, patients from higher socioeconomic families will be attracted to such hospitals, as will doctors with better qualifications. (The correlation coefficient between employees per bed and the family income of the patient is 0.11.) To inquire whether such doctor-patient interaction takes place, and if so, what effect such interactions have on hospital use, an interaction term was formed between the number of employees per bed and an income variable, and its effects on hospital use were examined. The results, however, were not enlightening.

The variables selected to represent hospital characteristics appear to have been well chosen. Regression analysis of the effects on hospital use of hospital dummy variables shows significant interhospital differences in hospital use, but in terms of explaining variations in hospital use among individual patients, the twenty-one hospital dummy variables are about as successful as ten variables representing hospital characteristics.

Patient Characteristics and Hospital Use

Patient characteristics as represented by fifteen to seventeen variables have much more success in explaining the variations in hospital use by individual patients than hospital characteristics as represented by eight variables. (The new R^2 range is 0.187 to 0.207 for unadjusted hospital use measures; 0.031 to 0.051 for the adjusted measures. See Tables 5-2 and 5-3.) This seems to be attributable to the fact that demographic and socioeconomic characteristics of individual patients as represented by fifteen to seventeen variables are more important in shaping the basis of doctor-patient interactions, and thereby in determining the amount and type of hospital care provided individual patients, than hospital characteristics. Since our model hypothesizes that hospital use is determined by doctor-patient interactions, patient characteristics that reflect patients' attitudes and expectations are expected to influence those interactions in a more important way than environmental and institutional factors (as represented by hospital characteristics) within which these interactions take place.

Turning to the separate effects on hospital use of specific patient characteristics, the most obvious and important ones are those of demographic variables. As expected, each patient age category received a greater amount of hospital care than all younger patient categories, no matter how hospital use was measured. The differences in hospital use by age are smaller when the adjusted (for diagnoses) measures of the amount of hospital care are used than when unadjusted measures are used. This is to be expected: older patients in general have more

TABLE 5-2

Patient Characteristics and Hospital Use, Unadjusted for Differences in Diagnoses (n = 8986) Double Log

Patient Characteristics	Length of Stay, Unadjusted		Total Services, Unadjusted		Total Bill, Unadjusted	
	b Coefficient	SE	b Coefficient	SE	b Coefficient	SE
Income	−0.0387	0.0234	−0.0310	0.0240	−0.0200	0.0208
Education[c]	0.0889[b]	0.0203	0.0099	0.0208	0.0243	0.0184
Race composition[d]	−0.0182[b]	0.0053	−0.0065	0.0054	−0.0084	0.0047
Method of payment						
Patient						
Service (free)	0.0723[b]	0.0165	0.1252[b]	0.0170	0.0836[b]	0.0150
Blue Cross	0.0438[b]	0.0131	0.0841[b]	0.0135	0.0467[b]	0.0117
Commercial insurance	0.0422[b]	0.0157	0.0711[b]	0.0162	0.0355[a]	0.0139
Government	0.1595[b]	0.0252	0.0741[b]	0.0259	0.1009[b]	0.0226
Unpaid or writeoff	0.0956[b]	0.0253	0.1364[b]	0.0260	0.0903[b]	0.0225
Employment status						
Unemployed or not stated	—		—		—	
Employed	0.0103	0.0102	0.0715[b]	0.0105	0.0075	0.0091
Living arrangement						
Living with others	—		—		—	
Living alone	0.0448[b]	0.0124	0.0098	0.0128	0.0191	0.0110

(continued)

(TABLE 5-2 concluded)

Room accommodation						
Ward	—	—	—	—	—	—
Semiprivate	—	—	—	—	0.0779b	0.0083
Private	—	—	—	—	0.1082b	0.0126
Age						
0–19 years	−0.4751b	0.0132	−0.4278b	0.0136	−0.4208b	0.0118
20–44 years	−0.2982b	0.0123	−0.3533b	0.0126	−0.2597b	0.0110
45–64 years	−0.0871	0.0127	−0.1025b	0.0130	−0.0821b	0.0113
65+ years	—	—	—	—	—	—
Race						
White	−0.0187	0.0125	−0.0438b	0.0128	−0.0271a	0.0111
Nonwhite	—	—	—	—	—	—
Sex						
Male	−0.0000	0.0086	0.0403b	0.0088	0.0034	0.0077
Female	—	—	—	—	—	—
a-constant	1.1153		1.2418		2.6357	
R-SQ	0.20315b (F = 152.5)		0.18810b (F = 138.6)		0.20829b (F = 138.5)	
Adjusted R-SQ	0.20182 (DF = 8971)		0.18675 (DF = 8971)		0.20679 (DF = 8969)	

a Significant at the 5 per cent level.
b Significant at the 1 per cent level.
c Per cent of population with less than eight years of schooling reported in census tract.
d Per cent of nonwhite population reported in census tract.

TABLE 5-3

Patient Characteristics and Hospital Use, Adjusted for Differences in Diagnoses ($n = 8986$) Double Log

Patient Characteristics	Length of Stay, Adjusted		Total Services, Adjusted		Total Bill, Adjusted	
	b Coefficient	SE	b Coefficient	SE	b Coefficient	SE
Income	−0.0447[a]	0.0214	−0.0498[a]	0.0196	−0.0224	0.0188
Education[c]	0.0738[b]	0.0186	0.0075	0.0170	0.0196	0.0167
Race composition[d]	−0.0114[a]	0.0048	−0.0045	0.0044	−0.0019	0.0042
Method of payment						
Patient						
Service (free)	0.0268	0.0151	0.0076[b]	0.0139	0.0308[a]	0.0136
Blue Cross	0.0082	0.0120	−0.0090	0.0110	0.0127	0.0106
Commercial insurance	0.0233	0.0144	0.0037	0.0132	0.0158	0.0127
Government	0.0914[b]	0.0231	0.0634[b]	0.0212	0.0442[a]	0.0205
Unpaid or writeoff	0.0481[a]	0.0232	0.0588[b]	0.0212	0.0398	0.0205
Employment status						
Unemployed or not stated	—		—		—	
Employed	−0.0215[a]	0.0094	0.0039	0.0086	−0.0167[a]	0.0082
Living arrangement						
Living with others	—		—		—	
Living alone	0.0242[a]	0.0114	−0.0119	0.0104	0.0041	0.0100

(continued)

(TABLE 5-3 concluded)

Room accommodation						
Ward	—	—	—	—	—	—
Semiprivate	—	—	—	—	0.0400[b]	0.0076
Private	—	—	—	—	0.0933[b]	0.0114
Age						
0–19 years	−0.1742[b]	0.0121	−0.1265[b]	0.0111	−0.1672[b]	0.0107
20–44 years	−0.0806[b]	0.0113	−0.0520[b]	0.0103	−0.0819[b]	0.0099
45–64 years	−0.0375[b]	0.0116	−0.0145	0.0106	−0.0362[b]	−0.0102
65+ years	—	—	—	—	—	—
Race						
White	−0.0032	0.0114	−0.0193	0.0104	−0.0111	0.0100
Nonwhite	—	—	—	—	—	—
Sex						
Male	−0.0466[b]	0.0079	−0.0061	0.0072	−0.0289[b]	0.0070
Female	—	—	—	—	—	—
a-constant	0.1205		0.1587		0.0412	
R-SQ	0.04574[b]	(F = 28.7)	0.03265[b]	(F = 20.2)	0.05312[b]	(F = 29.6)
Adjusted R-SQ	0.04415	(DF = 8971)	0.03103	(DF = 8971)	0.05132	(DF = 8969)

[a] Significant at 5 per cent level.
[b] Significant at 1 per cent level.
[c] Per cent of population with less than eight years of schooling reported in census tract.
[d] Per cent of nonwhite population reported in census tract.

serious illnesses than younger patients; to the extent to which adjusting for diagnoses eliminates the differences in hospital use due to differences in types of illnesses in different age groups, age differences in hospital use would diminish when adjusted measures are used.

The *b* coefficients of the sex variable show that proportionately more female patients are treated for less serious illnesses, but when treated for the same illnesses, they stay hospitalized longer, receive greater numbers of special services, and are charged more than male patients.

As expected, childbearing and other exclusively female conditions appear to be the principal reason more women are treated for less serious illnesses. Female patients whose principal diagnoses were listed as "delivery without complications" stayed, on the average, 5.7 days, compared with 9.1 days for all female patients, and these patients accounted for 19 per cent of all female patients discharged from hospitals. When the average lengths of stay are compared between sexes after the so-called female illnesses are excluded, female patients stay hospitalized about the same lengths of time (10.4 days) as male patients (10.3 days).

As for the variations in hospital use by race, whether the measures of hospital use are adjusted for differences in diagnoses or not, nonwhite patients stay longer, receive greater numbers of special services, and are charged more than white patients. The causes of this are difficult to theorize about because race and socioeconomic variables are intertwined in such a complex manner as to make the job of disentanglement very difficult. Not only is it readily assumed that proportionately more nonwhite patients are from families of low incomes, but also socioeconomic variables exert different influences on hospital use among whites and nonwhites.

There are significant differences in hospital use for given illnesses depending upon who pays the major portion of the hospital bill. When ranked from the greatest amount of use of hospital care to the least, the four major categories of patients by source of payment can be listed as government, free services, insurance, and patient. If the cure of an episode of illness is considered a transaction unit, the above variations in hospital use by method of payment can be interpreted as the result of the operation of price effect, because the order of ranking according to the relative amount of hospital use roughly corresponds, in reverse order, to that of the relative amount of out-of-pocket expenses incurred by the patient.

This, however, should not be explained away as simply a reflection of the price sensitivity of hospital use. The patient category as classified by method of payment may be related systematically to other factors, such as income, living arrangement, and employment status, and therefore a part of the difference in hospital use by method of payment may be attributable to these other factors.

The following list presents the correlation matrix among method of payment, employment status, and living arrangement:

	Employed	*Living Alone*
Patient	— .059	.031
Blue Cross	.105	— .085
Free service	— .180	.074
Government	— .088	.153

(The correlation coefficients are all statistically significant.) It is interesting to note that positive correlations with "employment" accompany negative correlations with "living alone."

For example, patients whose principal source of payment for hospital bills is themselves are likely to be unemployed and to live alone at home, while Blue Cross patients are likely to be employed and to live with someone else. Seen in this way, to the extent that the variables representing employment status and living arrangement failed to hold their effects on hospital use constant, "free service" and "government" patients may have used greater amounts of hospital care because they are likely to be unemployed and living alone at home.

The opportunity cost of time as represented by employment status has proved to be a choice-conditioning factor in hospital use. In an attempt to minimize the cost of time hospitalized, patients who are currently employed seek and succeed in receiving service-intensive care and thereby shorten the lengths of time they are hospitalized for given illnesses.

Since the employment status variable divides all patients into two categories only—those whose earnings foregone are nonzero and those whose earnings foregone are zero—a continuous variable representing the relative cost of time among those employed and those not employed is needed for a further examination of its effects on hospital use. The income variable in the context of the present analysis meets this need reasonably well, for the following reasons. First, the method-of-payment variable, which reflects the amount of out-of-pocket expenses regardless of size of hospital charges, neutralizes to a substantial extent the usual income effects operating through budget constraints. Second, to some extent the variable representing education severs the usual connection between income and taste.

The theory that, when method of payment, education, and the "cultural" factor are used as control variables, our income measure represents the cost of time can also conveniently explain the negative relationship between income and hospital use. Since it is hypothesized that hospital services are normal goods in terms of income elasticity of demand, and also because past studies show that high-income people use more hospital care than low-income people, the opposite result obtained in our study may be explained as the case where income measure represents mainly the cost of time. However, this leaves unresolved the important question of what the usual income effects on the consumption of hospital care are.

The hypothesis that, in the convalescent stage of illness, patients substitute general nursing care for inpatient hospital care if such care is available at home is supported by the relationship shown between the living-arrangment variable and hospital use. Those living alone seek and receive time-consuming care and thereby receive fewer special services and stay longer than those who have someone to look after them at home.

Interactions between Hospital Characteristics and Patient Characteristics, and Their Effects on Hospital Use

So far, we have explored two sets of relationships separately—one between patient characteristics and hospital use and the other between hospital characteristics and hospital use. The results indicate systematic variations in hospital use according to some of the variables representing patient characteristics and some of those representing hospital characteristics. This leaves the following question unresolved. Is the revealed relationship between *patient* characteristics and hospital use a reflection of different medical philosophies practiced by individual hospitals whose distinct modes of practice attract patients with distinct characteristics?

Looking at the relations from the other side, is the revealed relationship between *hospital* characteristics and hospital use attributable to the fact that patients at hospitals with different characteristics have different sets of expectations and demands? In this case, variations in hospital use by hospital characteristics merely reflect the responses to these different expectations and demands of patients.

Our hypothesis is that the answers to both questions are affirmative. Patients with certain characteristics choose hospitals with certain characteristics, and therefore patient and hospital characteristics are interrelated in their effects on hospital use. In analyzing the factors influencing hospital use, hospital characteristics could be treated as a reflection of patient characteristics, and vice versa. To test this hypothesis, various interaction terms between the variables representing patient characteristics and those for hospital characteristics were formed, and their effects on use examined.

Of the interaction terms whose relationships with hospital use were analyzed, several seemed to provide new insights; these are presented in Tables 5-4 and 5-5.

The data support the theory that hospital and patient characteristics are significantly interrelated. The correlation matrix constructed between thirteen variables representing patient characteristics and nine variables representing hospital characteristics shows that, with a few exceptions, correlations are statistically significant (Table 5-6).

A comparison of adjusted R^2's (the proportions of the variations in hospital use explained by the variables inserted in the regressions) among various regressions lends additional support to this theory. When variables representing hospital characteristics and those representing patient characteristics are combined and inserted into a single regression equation, there is only small improvement in the adjusted R^2, from 0.204 for the regression with variables representing patient characteristics only, and 0.035 for the regression with those representing hospital characteristics only, to 0.232.

More important, forming interaction terms between the two sets of variables enables us to sharpen our point of inquiry about specific hypotheses on the various relationships between individual variables chosen and hospital use. For example, our inquiry on how the method of payment affects hospital use is aided by forming an interaction term between the variables representing method of payment and occupancy rate. This enables us to ask what kind of hospital services consumers receive when they have a strong incentive to minimize hospital charges and hospitals are pressed for empty beds.

As shown by their b coefficients, the interaction terms between the variables representing the method of payment and occupancy rate have the same effects on hospital use as those of the method of payment variables alone. As before, patients whose hospital bills are paid by the government use the most hospital care, those whose costs are borne by individual hospitals as free services are next, insurance-paid patients are third, and patients who pay their own bills use the least hospital care.

What is gained by the interaction terms is that the differences in

TABLE 5-4

Interaction Terms Between Patient Characteristics and Hospital Characteristics, and Their Relationships to Hospital Use, Unadjusted for Differences in Diagnoses (n = 8986) Double Log

Patient and Hospital Characteristics	Length of Stay, Unadjusted		Total Services, Unadjusted		Total Bill, Unadjusted	
	b Coefficient	SE	b Coefficient	SE	b Coefficient	SE
Method of payment × occupancy rate						
Patient × occupancy rate						
Patient × occupancy	—	—	—	—	—	—
Service × occupancy	0.0958[b]	0.0198	0.1459[b]	0.0202	0.0436[a]	0.0176
Blue Cross × occupancy	0.0590[b]	0.0152	0.1104[b]	0.0155	0.0578[b]	0.0134
Commercial × occupancy	0.0607[b]	0.0189	0.1140[b]	0.0193	0.0437[b]	0.0168
Other insurance × occupancy	0.0788[b]	0.0334	0.0169	0.0341	−0.0018	0.0296
Government × occupancy	0.1716[b]	0.0294	0.0605[a]	0.0301	0.0360	0.0261
Other × occupancy	0.1074[b]	0.0298	0.1435[b]	0.0304	0.0463	0.0264
Beds × occupancy	0.1569[b]	0.0204	0.0981[b]	0.0208	0.2004[b]	0.0181
Personnel per bed × income	−0.0640[b]	0.0172	−0.0097	0.0195	0.0148	0.0170
Occupancy × outpatient clinic × living with others	−0.0472[b]	0.0123	−0.0825[b]	0.0126	−0.0180	0.0109

(continued)

(TABLE 5-4 concluded)

Race × room accommodation	-0.0037	0.0154	-0.0140	0.0168	-0.0169	0.0145
Internship × residency × nursing	-0.0051	0.0108	0.0595[b]	0.0110	-0.0309[b]	0.0096
Income × employed	-0.0000	0.0000	0.0000[b]	0.0000	0.0000	0.0000
Race × per cent nonwhite	0.0005	0.0019	0.0071[b]	0.0020	0.0029	0.0017
Age						
0–19 years	—	—	—	—	—	—
20–44 years	0.1752[b]	0.0105	0.0733[b]	0.0110	0.1678[b]	0.0035
45–64 years	0.3829[b]	0.0117	0.3098[b]	0.0120	0.3458[b]	0.0104
65+ years	0.4712[b]	0.0131	0.4039[b]	0.0134	0.4297[b]	0.0115
Male	0.0031	0.0084	0.0453[b]	0.0086	-0.0046	0.0075
a-constant	0.4188		0.4874		1.6646	
Multiple R	0.45781		0.45121		0.46060	
R-SQ	0.20959[b]	(F = 139.9)	0.20359[b]	(F = 134.9)	0.21215[b]	(F = 142.1)
Adjusted R-SQ	0.20809	(DF = 8964)	0.20208		0.21065	

[a] Significant at the 5 per cent level.
[b] Significant at the 1 per cent level.

TABLE 5-5

Interaction Terms Between Patient Characteristics and Hospital Characteristics, and Their Relationships to Hospital Use, Adjusted for Differences in Diagnoses (n = 8986) Double Log

Patient and Hospital Characteristics	Length of Stay, Adjusted		Total Services, Adjusted		Total Bill, Adjusted	
	b Coefficient	SE	b Coefficient	SE	b Coefficient	SE
Method of payment × occupancy rate						
Patient × occupancy	—	—	—	—	—	—
Service × occupancy	0.0354	0.0182	0.0839[b]	0.0165	−0.0031	0.0159
Blue Cross × occupancy	0.0134	0.0139	0.0065	0.0126	0.0119	0.0122
Commercial × occupancy	0.0357[a]	0.0174	0.0342[a]	0.0157	0.0172	0.0152
Other insurance × occupancy	0.0354	0.0307	−0.0333	0.0278	−0.0203	0.0269
Government × occupancy	0.0926[b]	0.0270	0.0596[a]	0.0245	−0.0102	0.0237
Other × occupancy	0.0515	0.0273	0.0515[a]	0.0247	0.0024	0.0239
Beds × occupancy	0.1178[b]	0.0187	0.1553[b]	0.0170	0.1725[b]	0.0164
Personnel per bed × income	−0.0697[b]	0.0176	−0.0195	0.0159	0.0062	0.0154
Occupancy × outpatient clinic × living with others	−0.0104	0.0113	−0.0234[a]	0.0102	0.0104	0.0099

(continued)

(TABLE 5-5 concluded)

Race × room accommodation	0.0175	0.0150	0.0273[a]	0.0136	0.0046	0.0132
Internship × residency × nursing	-0.0087	0.0097	0.0246[b]	0.0090	-0.0304[b]	0.0087
Income × employed	-0.0000[b]	0.0000	-0.0000	0.0000	-0.0000	0.0000
Race × per cent nonwhite	-0.0029	-1.6277	-0.0003	0.0016	-0.0004	0.0015
Age						
0-19 years	—	—	—	—	—	—
20-44 years	0.0919[b]	0.0099	0.0694[b]	0.0090	0.0850[b]	0.0087
45-64 years	0.1343[b]	0.0107	0.0973[b]	0.0097	0.1337[b]	0.0094
65+ years	0.1749[b]	0.0120	0.1115[b]	0.0109	0.1764[b]	0.0105
Male	-0.0452[b]	0.0077	-0.0052	0.0070	-0.0353[b]	0.0068
a-constant	-0.1953		-0.4399		-0.6158	
Multiple R	0.22512		0.23725		0.24500	
R-SQ	0.05068[b]	(F = 28.2)	0.05629[b]	(F = 31.5)	0.06002[b]	(F = 33.7)
Adjusted R-SQ	0.04888	(DF = 8969)	0.05450		0.05824	

[a] Significant at the 5 per cent level.
[b] Significant at the 1 per cent level.

TABLE 5-6

Correlation Matrix: Relationships Between Patient Characteristics and Hospital Characteristics ($n = 8986$)

Patient and Hospital Characteristics	Occupancy Rate	Facilities Weighted	Intern Program	Presence of Nursing School	Employees per Bed	Payroll Total Expenses	Number of Personnel	Presence of Home-care Program	Presence of Out-patient Clinic
Income	0.0738	0.0001	0.0008	0.0315	0.1145	-0.0221	0.0003	0.1001	-0.0730
Housing[a]	-0.0520	0.0505	0.0065	0.0036	-0.0628	0.0548	-0.0020	-0.0689	0.0860
Education[b]	-0.0854	0.0350	-0.0077	-0.0317	-0.1198	0.0121	-0.0171	-0.1100	0.1001
Racial composition[c]	-0.0930	0.0739	-0.0324	0.0097	0.0757	0.0282	-0.0204	0.0338	0.0693
Race									
White = 1	0.1314	-0.0943	0.0474	0.0157	-0.0668	-0.0194	-0.0101	-0.0777	-0.0667
Method of payment									
Free service dummy	-0.0820	0.0675	-0.0196	0.0016	0.0713	0.0501	0.0280	-0.0134	0.0584
Patient dummy	0.0128	-0.0049	-0.0102	-0.0136	0.0196	0.0026	0.0042	-0.0022	-0.0140
Blue Cross dummy	0.0240	-0.0363	-0.0022	-0.0249	-0.0151	-0.0346	-0.0386	0.0515	-0.0115
Commercial insurance dummy	0.0007	-0.0534	-0.0279	-0.0308	-0.0274	-0.0212	-0.0057	-0.0331	-0.0442
Government dummy	0.0103	-0.0033	0.0173	0.0229	-0.0167	-0.0089	0.0180	-0.0152	-0.0155
Marital status									
Married = 1	-0.0376	0.0307	-0.0024	-0.0140	0.0006	0.0057	0.0099	0.0422	-0.0158
Employment status									
Employed = 1	0.0940	0.0295	0.0988	0.1091	-0.0243	0.0243	0.0247	0.0156	-0.0283
Living arrangement									
Living alone = 1	0.0293	0.0333	0.0516	0.0701	0.0024	0.0213	0.0147	-0.0184	0.0022

Note: $r \geq .0206$, significant at .05 confidence level.
 $r \geq .0272$, significant at .01 confidence level.

[a] Per cent of substandard units reported in census tract.
[b] Per cent of population with less than eight years of schooling reported in census tract.
[c] Per cent of nonwhite population reported in census tract.

hospital use according to who pays the major portion of the hospital bill are crystallized. Note that in most cases the magnitudes of *b* coefficients which show the differences in the amount of hospital use from that by those who pay the bill themselves have increased.

This indicates that, to the extent that the amount of out-of-pocket expenses incurred by each patient represents the price of the cure of an episode of illness, the price sensitivity of hospital use increases when the hospital has fewer empty beds. It has been pointed out, however, that the relationship between the method-of-payment variable and hospital use cannot be simply interpreted as price elasticity of demand for hospital care because of intercorrelation between method-of-payment variables and those representing income, living arrangements, employment status, et cetera. Unfortunately, forming interaction terms between the method-of-payment variables and those other variables and examining their effects on hospital use yielded no new useful information.

Previously, the opportunity cost of time was measured by whether the patient was currently employed. Since this employment status variable divides all patients into two categories only, an interaction term was formed between employment status and income variables to examine how the costs of time among those who are employed, as measured by their family incomes, affected hospital use. As expected, the regression analyses showed that the greater the opportunity cost of time as measured by the interaction term, the shorter the length of stay.

In addition, since the housewife is not employed and yet her cost of time is not zero in terms of housework foregone, another interaction term was formed among the variables representing income, employment status, and sex of the patient. Regressing this interaction term against hospital use showed that high-income male patients currently employed seek hospitalization for the treatment of more serious illnesses than others, but that, once hospitalized, they stay for shorter periods of time for given illnesses by seeking service-intensive care to minimize the cost of time hospitalized. (This regression is not reproduced here.)

It has been hypothesized that the extent to which the costs of time affect hospital use depends on out-of-pocket expenses. In testing this hypothesis we have gained little enlightenment through the use of interaction terms such as that between the cost-of-time variable and the per cent of the hospital bill paid by the patient. Therefore, in analyzing the effect of the cost of time on hospital use, the out-of-pocket expenses are represented by the dummy variables showing the method of payment, and they are used as control variables, thus holding their effect on hospital use constant.

It has been shown that, for given illnesses, patients living alone stay hospitalized longer than those living with others at home, indicating that in the convalescent stage of illness patients substitute hospital care for general nursing care if such care is available at home. In order to determine the extent to which such substitutions take place and how this affects inpatient hospital use, an interaction term was formed among the variables representing occupancy rate, the presence of an outpatient clinic, and living arrangements.

This enabled us to ask whether—if the hospital has an outpatient clinic which facilitates ambulatory treatment, the patient has somebody to take care of him at home, and the hospital is pressed for empty beds—the doctors will discharge the patient as early as possible to alleviate the bed shortage by substituting inpatient care for outpatient care at outpatient clinics and at home. The result shows that such substitutions do take place under these conditions and, therefore, the patient stays a shorter period of time and a relatively lower number of special services are administered while he is hospitalized. This is a case where doctor-patient interaction reinforces the expectations and motivations of both.

It has been shown that patients treated at hospitals which have graduate medical training programs receive more hospital care than those treated at hospitals without such programs and that patients in hospitals with nursing schools receive more service-intensive care and stay shorter periods than those in hospitals without nursing schools. In order to investigate the relationship between training programs and hospital use by the patients, an interaction term was formed among variables representing the presence of an internship program, a residency program, and a nursing school, and its effects on hospital use was examined. The result indicates that the patients at the hospitals with all three training programs receive service-intensive care and stay shorter periods for given illnesses.

An explanation for this finding was sought in the hypothesis that teaching hospitals are usually prestigious and that they attract doctors and patients with certain characteristics. Therefore, the fact that the patients in these hospitals receive a different type and amount of care may simply reflect specific types of doctor-patient interactions. This hypothesis was tested by forming an interaction term between the variables representing the presence of medical training programs and the family incomes of patients. This crude measure of doctor-patient interactions yielded no new insight into the validity of the hypothesis. (In a similar vein, the distinct patterns of patient care in hospitals with different numbers of facilities were examined by forming an interaction term between income and weighted number of facilities. The results again provided no new insights.)

Another hypothesis tested was that more special services are provided to patients in the hospitals with training programs because more tests are conducted there to establish normal results for teaching purposes. Since most of these tests for teaching purposes are administered to ward patients, this hypothesis was tested by forming an interaction term between the variables representing the presence of graduate medical education programs, race, and ward room accommodation and then by examining its effects on hospital use. The results showed that non-white patients in wards receive a significantly greater number of special services than white patients in semiprivate or private rooms.

It has been observed that nonwhite patients use more hospital care than white patients, but there is a negative relationship between racial composition of neighborhood and hospital use. This conflicting result poses a problem of interpretation. Is this conflicting relationship attributable to the difference in the neighborhood effect and the racial effect on hospital use?

One may point out that nonwhites in predominantly white neighborhoods behave differently from those in predominantly nonwhite neighborhoods. Not much use can be made of this theory here because, in view of the prevailing racial pattern of residential districts, it is doubtful that the racial-composition variable has succeeded in isolating neighborhood effects on hospital use. (The data show that the correlation coefficient between the race variable white $= 1$ and the racial-composition variable is 0.58.) On the other hand, the fact that both race and racial-composition variables have significant b coefficients in terms of t ratios indicates that the multicollinearity problem is not serious. Analysis of an interaction term formed between race and racial-composition variables and its relationship to hospital use showed that nonwhite patients from predominantly nonwhite neighborhoods were hospitalized for more serious illnesses than white patients, but for given illness they stayed shorter periods and paid less than white patients in white neighborhoods. This confirms our a priori reasoning about behavior patterns of the nonwhite patients, many of whom probably are lower on the socioeconomic scale.

The reasons for this observed relationship of the interaction term between race and racial composition vis-à-vis hospital use were sought in a possible correlation between race and income and that between race and education, and in their effects on hospital use. Income and education were examined because they are the most obvious causes of differences in the behavior patterns of white and nonwhite patients.

The correlation matrix presented below indicates that, as expected, white patients have higher incomes, more education, and better jobs than nonwhite patients.

Race (white = 1; nonwhite = 0)

Income	.266
Education	
(the lack of)	− .365
Occupation	.139

(Education is represented by the per cent of the population twenty-five years old or older who had less than eight years of schooling; occupation, by the per cent of the population who had managerial or professional jobs.) However, when an interaction term is formed between race and income and another between race and education, and their effects on hospital use are examined, no new insights are obtained.

The occupancy rate was negatively related to hospital use. This relationship cannot be taken seriously, however, because it is insignificant. It seems to be attributable to the fact that occupancy rate is an unsatisfactory variable to represent the relative scarcity of empty beds because occupancy rate is systematically related to number of beds regardless of the pressure of demand for these beds. (The correlation coefficient between the number of beds and occupancy rate is 0.19.) Thus, when the availability of beds is represented by an interaction term between occupancy rate and the number of beds in other regressions, it has a positive and significant relationship with all six measures of hospital use. This provides one more piece of evidence that an increase in supply of beds will, ceteris paribus, result in some increase in hospital use.

6

An Economic Analysis of Variations in Medical Expenses and Work-Loss Rates

Morris Silver

1. OBJECTIVES AND ORGANIZATION

This paper employs a number of the standard tools of economic analysis to explore unpublished data on the medical expenses and work-loss days due to illness or injury of currently employed persons. Section 2 deals with the data, statistical techniques, and variables employed in the study. The primary objective of Section 3 is to estimate elasticities of demand for medical care (totally and by type) with respect to family income. Knowledge of these elasticities should contribute to more accurate forecasts of the demand for medical care and aid in the formulation of policy-related judgments concerning the equity of the current distribution of medical services.

Like earlier studies of the demand for medical care[1] which have

NOTE: This paper appeared previously in Herbert E. Klarman (ed.), *Empirical Studies in Health Economics; Proceedings of the Second Conference on the Economics of Health,* Baltimore, Johns Hopkins Press, 1970, pp. 121–40.

This research was carried out at the National Bureau of Economic Research and was supported in part by grants from the Commonwealth Fund and by the National Center for Health Services Research and Development, Grant 1P01CH00374–01. I am indebted to Richard Auster, Gary Becker, Michael Grossman, Irving Leveson, Jacob Mincer, Kong-Kyun Ro, and, most of all, to Victor R. Fuchs for many helpful comments. Special thanks are due Mrs. Geraldine A. Gleeson, Chief, Analysis and Reports Branch, Division of Health Interview Statistics, National Center for Health Statistics, United States Public Health Service, for providing me with the work-loss and medical expense data.

[1] Paul J. Feldstein and Ruth Severson, "The Demand for Medical Care," *Report of the Commission on the Cost of Medical Care,* Chicago, American Medical Association, 1964, pp. 57–76; Grover Wirick and Robin Barlow, "The Economic and Social Determinants of the Demand for Health Services," in *The Economics of Health and Medical Care,* ed. S. J. Axelrod, Ann Arbor, The

utilized other bodies of data, the present study utilizes data on medical expenses to measure the amount of care received. Expense data are useful because, unlike the available physical measures, they reflect not only the quantity but the quality of medical care. On the other hand, the use of expense data creates a number of problems (e.g., free care) which are given detailed consideration in Section 3.

Unlike many previous studies, this study makes use of grouped or "ecological" data. The use of average incomes to estimate income elasticities which describe individual behavior can be justified in two ways. First, grouped data should minimize "simultaneous-equation bias." The individual correlation between income and medical care will reflect not only the effect of income on the amount of medical care demanded but also the effect of health on income. This problem would be more severe for individual than for grouped data because individual health is affected not only by differences in "erratic" factors among groups but by intragroup variations in such factors. Second, measurement errors (including transitory influences) in individual incomes would lead to underestimates of regression coefficients even if these errors were not correlated with the true (or long-run) individual incomes.[2] Errors of this type often cancel out in grouped data.

One of the important innovations of Section 3 is the inclusion of the earnings rate with family income in the regressions. This allows empirically for the previously ignored possibility that higher-income individuals may need more medical care or use less patient–time-intensive methods of dealing with their medical problems.

The mortality rate has been the most widely used measure of health for many years, but the recent growth of quantitative interest in the determinants of health status has sharply increased the demand for more flexible measures. One of the most promising alternative measures

---

University of Michigan Press, 1964, pp. 95–125; Paul J. Feldstein and W. John Carr, "The Effect of Income on Medical Care Spending," *Proceedings of the Social Statistics Section of the American Statistical Association,* 1964, pp. 93–105. For useful summaries, references to the literature, and discussions of many of the relevant issues in the theory and empirical application of the demand for medical services, see Herbert E. Klarman, *The Economics of Health,* New York, Columbia University Press, 1965, chap. 2; Paul J. Feldstein, "Research on the Demand for Health Services," *Milbank Memorial Fund Quarterly* 44, July 1966, pp. 128–62; and Jerome Rothenberg, "Comment," *Proceedings of the Social Statistics Section of the American Statistical Association,* 1964, pp. 109–10. See also Part III of this volume.

[2] J. Johnston, *Econometric Methods,* New York, McGraw-Hill Book Co., 1963, pp. 148–50.

of health is the work-loss rate due to illness or injury. Section 4 attempts to test the validity of using the work-loss rate as a measure of health by ascertaining whether variations in work-loss rates reflect differences in the degree to which individuals can afford to lose income or in the amounts that would be lost, and, if so, the extent to which they do so. The principal findings of the study are summarized in Section 5.

2. DATA, VARIABLES, AND STATISTICAL TECHNIQUES

The medical expense and work-loss data analyzed are drawn from the National Health Survey of the National Center for Health Statistics. These data, which are restricted to currently employed persons, are in the form of averages for each of twenty-four groups, by regions (Northeast, North Central, South, and West), age group (17–44, 45–64, and 65 and over), and sex.

The information was obtained through household health interviews and mail-in questionnaires left after completion of the interviews. The averages for medical expenses are based on a sample of about 71,000 persons from 22,000 households and include all medical bills paid, or to be paid, by the ill person, his family or friends, and any part paid by insurance. The average work-loss rates are based upon a sample of 134,000 persons from 42,000 households. The expense data refer to the twelve months prior to the interview period of July 1, 1962–December 31, 1962, while the work-loss data refer to the interview period July 1962–June 1963.[3]

The primary data utilized in the paper are shown in Table 6-1. The data for the quantitative independent variables are, of necessity, also in the form of averages for each of the twenty-four region-age-sex cells and refer to employed persons at work. However, those averages which refer to 1959 or 1960 are derived from a different sample than the medical expenses and work-loss rates, the 1-in-1,000 sample of the census of 1960.[4]

[3] For more detailed discussions of the work-loss and expense data, see U.S. Department of Health, Education, and Welfare, Public Health Service, National Center for Health Statistics, *Personal Health Expenses per Capita Annual Expenses, United States: July–December 1962,* Vital and Health Statistics, series 10, no. 27, Washington, D.C., 1966, and *Disability Days in the United States: July 1963–June 1964,* Vital and Health Statistics, series 10, no. 24, Washington, D.C., 1965.

[4] U.S. Department of Commerce, Bureau of the Census, *Census of Population and Housing, 1/1,000 and 1/10,000: Two National Samples of the Population of the United States,* Washington, D.C., 1960.

The more important variables employed in the multiple regressions of Sections 3 and 4 are listed below and discussed when appropriate.

TABLE 6-1

Selected Data on Medical Expenses and Days Lost from Work, by
Age Group and Sex

Region	Age Group	Sex	Average Medical Expenses per Currently Employed Person per Year (July–December 1962)	Average Days Lost due to Illness or Injury per Currently Employed Person per Year (July 1962–June 1963)
NE	17–44	M	$106.99	3.5
NE	45–64	M	175.12	7.1
NE	65 and over	M	228.89	8.2
NE	17–44	F	154.47	6.5
NE	45–64	F	193.81	8.7
NE	65 and over	F	269.79	6.4
NC	17–44	M	90.30	3.9
NC	45–64	M	161.00	6.9
NC	65 and over	M	190.45	10.6
NC	17–44	F	129.83	5.5
NC	45–64	F	181.17	6.7
NC	65 and over	F	163.53	5.4
S	17–44	M	95.50	5.4
S	45–64	M	156.92	9.8
S	65 and over	M	175.12	13.8
S	17–44	F	140.95	6.5
S	45–64	F	168.23	6.3
S	65 and over	F	142.09	7.1
W	17–44	M	114.59	4.8
W	45–64	M	192.37	6.2
W	65 and over	M	203.94	9.8
W	17–44	F	216.81	6.6
W	45–64	F	249.30	6.0
W	65 and over	F	183.05	7.5

Dependent Variables:

Y_1, total medical expense per currently employed person per year

Y_2, hospital expense per currently employed person per year

Y_3, medicine expense per currently employed person per year

Y_4, doctor expense per currently employed person per year

Y_5, dentist expense per currently employed person per year

Y_6, days lost from work due to illness or injury per currently employed person per year

Independent Variables:[5]

Average weekly earnings are obtained by dividing mean total earnings for a given cell by its mean number of weeks worked. Earnings per day are estimated by dividing the above quotient by 5; the resulting dollar figure is multiplied by mean work-loss days in the cell to obtain the value of lost time, which is then added to X_{1u}.

X_1,　adjusted mean total family income for employed persons at work who are in families

X_{1u}, unadjusted mean total family income for employed persons at work who are in families

X_{1d}, 0 if adjusted mean total family income for employed persons at work in families (X_1) is below its median value; the actual value of X_1 when it is above its median

X_2,　0 for female, 1 for male

X_3,　region: 0 for non-South, 1 for South

X_4,　age: 0 for 17–44, 1 for 45–64, 2 for 65 and over

X_3 and X_4 are the primary measures of region and age utilized in the study. The forms of these variables are derived from a priori considerations and from a desire to conserve degrees of freedom, to limit multicollinearity problems, and to avoid exhausting the sample space. The age variable is the most controversial, but it is important to note that the possibility that its use biases the coefficients of the economic variables upon which our interest centers is lessened by the use of a variety of regression forms. However, as an additional precaution, key results are checked by replacing X_3 with:

X_5, age: 1 if age 17–44, 0 otherwise

and

X_6, age: 1 if age 45–64, 0 otherwise

---

[5] The following midpoints were assumed for open-ended classes: total family income of employed persons at work in families (Item 60, Code X), $60,000; total earnings of employed persons at work (Item 39, Code X), $40,000; highest grade of school completed by employed persons at work (Item 26, Code X), 17.5 years.

X_7, mean highest grade of school completed by employed persons at work

X_8, percentage of employed persons at work residing in rural areas

X_9, percentage of employed persons at work residing outside SMSA's

X_{10}, percentage of employed persons at work who are married with spouse present

X_{11}, percentage of employed persons at work who are Negro

X_{12}, earnings per week worked of employed persons at work (estimated by dividing mean total earnings in 1959 for those with earnings by the mean number of weeks worked in 1959 by those who worked)

Since the relevant bodies of theory do not specify functional forms, both natural values and a logarithmic transformation are employed. Further, the regressions are run in both unweighted and weighted form, in which the weights are the square roots of the number of persons in each of the twenty-four region-age-sex cells. The use of weights is designed to achieve homoscedasticity and reduce the chances of errors in regression coefficients caused by large random errors in a small cell. However, unweighted regressions are run also because relevant information might be lost by the assignment of low weights to small but extreme cells (e.g., those for the 65-and-over age group).

3. REGRESSION ANALYSIS OF MEDICAL EXPENSES

The primary objective of this section is to estimate elasticities of demand for medical care with respect to command over goods and services. Amounts of medical services received are measured by the mean medical expenses of currently employed persons in a region-age-sex cell (Y_1–Y_5), while command over goods and services is measured by a cell's adjusted mean total family income for employed persons at work who are in families (X_1).

An important advantage of expense data is that they reflect both the quantity and quality of medical care, whereas the available physical measures (e.g., physician visits) reflect only the quantity. However, as in previous studies, the use of expenses gives rise to a number of difficulties. First there is the (probably minor) problem of "free" care which is received by some currently employed persons with very low incomes but is not included in the expense data. Second, medical care prices may be positively correlated with income because physicians charge the more affluent higher prices for given services, or because the more affluent are more likely to have health insurance and those covered by insurance are charged higher prices.[6] Third, and most important, when more affluent individuals are ill or undergoing preventive care, they attempt to maintain their customary living standards by purchasing amenities and complements to medical care such as private hospital rooms and "Park Avenue doctors." As a result, the medical expenses of the more affluent overstate the amount of medical care they have received.

The available data do not permit dealing with the last two problems. However, the purchase of amenities is probably most important in the case of hospital expense, and the data do permit the estimation of separate income elasticities for the various components of medical care.

As has been pointed out in Section 1, the use of mean incomes helps to minimize bias due to errors of measurement and simultaneous-equation problems. However, if variables not included in the statistical model reduced health in certain of our region-age-sex cells and resulted in higher medical expenses and lower family income, income elasticities would still be biased. In order to deal with this possibility, data for each region-age-sex cell on average earnings rates and work-loss days due to illness or injury were used to estimate the value of working time lost due to poor health. These estimates were added to the mean family income figure for each of the cells to secure "adjusted" mean total family income (X_1), which was utilized in the regressions.

Since higher-income individuals can afford to purchase more and better medical care and are unlikely to prefer purchases of other types of consumer goods when they are ill, and since it seems unlikely that most consumers regard the services provided by preventive medical care as lower-quality members of some broader family of services (as is margarine in the family of table fats), there is reason to expect the income elasticity to be positive. On the other hand, given appropriate assumptions about time preferences, it is possible that those with higher incomes might purchase more preventive care, resulting in lower average current expenses.[7] In the opinion of this writer the arguments suggest-

---

[6] These possibilities are mentioned by Victor R. Fuchs in his Comment in *The Economics of Health and Medical Care,* 1964, p. 126. It should be noted that the direction of the bias caused by a sliding scale of fees depends upon the elasticity of demand for medical care with respect to its price. If, as is generally assumed, demand is inelastic, a positive correlation between medical care prices and income would lead to overestimation of income elasticities.

[7] Wirick and Barlow, "The Economic and Social Determinants of the Demand for Health Services," p. 107.

ing a positive relationship are far stronger than those supporting a negative one, but in the final analysis the issue must be resolved by the data.

Previous empirical studies indicate that the income elasticity is positive and somewhat below unity. The latter magnitude is a useful benchmark because of the "necessity" character of much, if not most, medical expenditure. If we continue to think in terms of the "degree of necessity," it seems reasonable to expect the income elasticity of dentist expense to be relatively high and that of hospital expense to be relatively low. This hypothesis receives support from the findings of Feldstein and Severson[8] and is reexamined in the present study.

Because of their intrinsic interest and to avoid biased estimation of the income elasticity, a number of additional independent variables are included in the regressions. Dummy variables measuring age, sex, and region are utilized because they may reflect differences in physiological or psychological needs for medical care,[9] or perhaps in its cost. Later in the analysis, the percentage rural, the percentage living outside SMSA's, the percentage Negro, and measures of marital status and education are included in the regressions. In the final phase the earnings rate is introduced. The studies cited above suggest that being younger and better educated lowers expenses, while being female raises them. The results of the regressions are presented in Table 6–2.

Regressions 1–4 show that whatever the form employed, the coefficient of income is positive and statistically significant at conventional levels.[10] The estimated income elasticities of demand for medical services, which range from 1.4 to 2.0, are quite high in comparison with those observed in previous studies.

The inclusion of bills paid by insurance in the expense data, taken together with a positive correlation between family income and the amount of health insurance (whether directly paid for by the family

---

[8] See "The Demand for Medical Care."

[9] Wirick and Barlow, pp. 101, 104.

[10] X_{1d} was introduced into the regressions in order to ascertain whether the effect of income varies with its level. It was found that the coefficient of this variable, which measures the difference in the effect of income in the range below its median from that in the range above its median, fluctuates in sign and is statistically insignificant.

In practice, the use of "adjusted" income did not matter very much; when regression 4 was rerun utilizing unadjusted income (X_{1u}), the income elasticity was 2.04 and its computed t value was 5.44, while the adjusted coefficient of determination was 0.89.

or by third parties), may help to explain the above discrepancy. Along the same lines, some studies include insurance coverage as an independent variable, which causes income elasticities to be underestimated since, to a large extent, insurance coverage is a positive function of income. Unfortunately, the data at my disposal do not permit quantitative statements of the role of these factors. Another possibility which is difficult to test is that preventive care, which is probably more income-elastic than care of the curative variety, comprises a larger fraction of total medical expenses for the currently employed population than for the population as a whole.

Since the LW form showed the strongest results, sole reliance was now placed upon it. The next step taken was to replace X_4 by the less demanding age variables X_5 and X_6 (see regression 5).[11] Since the coefficients of these variables were found to be statistically significant, to increase the unadjusted coefficient of determination slightly, and to raise the estimated income elasticity from 2.0 to 2.5, it was decided to retain them in the succeeding regressions. Regressions 6–9 are for the separate components of medical expense and show the relative magnitudes of the income elasticities to be consistent with a priori considerations and previous empirical work—i.e., the income elasticities range from 1.8 for hospital expense to 3.2 for dentist expense.

The results for the other independent variables utilized in regressions 1–9 may be summarized as follows: Other things being equal, the proxy for the quantity of medical services is higher for females, Southerners, and older persons (with the exception of dental care) than for males, non-Southerners, and younger persons.[12] Some possible interpretations are (1) that younger persons and non-Southerners require less medical care because they are healthier than older persons and Southerners, and (2) that for physiological or psychological reasons females purchase more and/or more expensive medical care than males.

In regressions 10–14 some new independent variables are introduced one at a time into regressions for total expenses. The coefficients of the percentage rural (X_8) and the percentage outside SMSA's (X_9) are

---

[11] The coefficients of X_5 and X_6 show how much the level of the entire equation must be adjusted for the influence of the corresponding age groups; the influence of the age group sixty-five and over is reflected in the constant term of the equation.

[12] When X_4 is used in regressions 6–9 instead of X_5 and X_6, the ordering of income elasticities remains the same while the coefficients of X_4 are 0.15, 0.16, 0.08, and −0.04, respectively. The corresponding computed t values are 4.20, 11.67, 3.73, and −1.25, respectively.

TABLE 6-2
Regressions of Medical Expenses per Currently Employed Person per Year on Various Independent Variables for Twenty-four Region-Age-Sex Cells[a]

Regression No. (1)	Form of Regression[b] and Dependent Variable (2)	Regression Coefficient and Computed t Value (in Parentheses)[c]						Biased Coefficient of Determination and Unbiased Coefficient of Determination (in Parentheses) (9)
		Income (X_1) (3)	Sex (X_2) (4)	Region (X_3) (5)	Age (X_4) or Age (X_5) (6)	Age (X_6) (7)	$X_7 - X_{12}$ (8)	
1	NU$_w$ Tot. exp. (Y_1)	0.03 (3.42)[e]	−34.90 (−3.01)[e]	33.50 (1.45)	37.19 (5.27)[e]			.70 (.63)
2	NW Tot. exp. (Y_1)	0.03 (4.32)[e]	−43.95 (−6.15)[e]	47.33 (2.92)[e]	36.10 (5.38)[e]			.88 (.85)
3	LU$_w$ Tot. exp. (Y_1)	1.55 (4.01)[e]	−0.10 (−3.61)[e]	0.12 (2.04)	0.11 (6.24)[e]			.75 (.70)
4	LW Tot. exp. (Y_1)	2.02 (5.61)[e]	−0.14 (−7.64)[e]	0.18 (4.16)[e]	0.11 (6.40)[e]			.91 (.90)
5	LW Tot. exp. (Y_1)	2.53 (5.38)[e]	−0.14 (−8.10)[e]	0.24 (4.35)[e]	−0.26 (−6.34)[e]	−0.18 (−3.79)[e]		.92 (.90)
6	LW Hos. exp. (Y_2)	1.82 (1.74)	−0.14 (−3.69)[e]	0.17 (1.43)	−0.32 (−3.56)[e]	−0.19 (−1.77)		.74 (.67)
7	LW Med. exp. (Y_3)	2.23 (5.62)[e]	−0.15 (−10.52)[e]	0.29 (6.16)[e]	−0.34 (−10.05)[e]	−0.20 (−4.93)[e]		.96 (.95)
8	LW Dr. exp. (Y_4)	2.88 (4.56)[e]	−0.15 (−6.42)[e]	0.29 (3.94)[e]	−0.21 (−4.04)[e]	−0.18 (−2.78)[d]		.86 (.82)
9	LW Den. exp. (Y_5)	3.19 (3.55)[e]	−0.13 (−3.75)[e]	0.22 (2.08)	0.04 (0.47)	−0.04 (−0.44)		.71 (.62)

(continued)

TABLE 6-2 (continued)

								R²
10	LW Tot. exp. (Y₁)	2.61 (5.47)ᵉ	−0.13 (−5.70)ᵉ	0.28 (4.11)ᵉ	−0.34 (−3.81)ᵉ	−0.22 (−3.58)ᵉ	[Ed. X₇] 0.74 (1.01)	.93 (.90)
11	LW Tot. exp. (Y₁)	2.39 (4.12)ᵉ	−0.13 (−5.24)ᵉ	0.24 (4.17)ᵉ	−0.26 (−6.19)ᵉ	−0.17 (−3.35)ᵉ	[% rural X₈] −0.05 (−0.43)	.92 (.90)
12	LW Tot. exp. (Y₁)	2.38 (4.16)ᵉ	−0.14 (−7.34)ᵉ	0.23 (4.08)ᵉ	−0.25 (−6.21)ᵉ	−0.18 (−3.50)ᵉ	[% out. SMSA X₉] −0.04 (−0.47)	.93 (.90)
13	LW Tot. exp. (Y₁)	2.35 (5.30)ᵉ	−0.20 (−6.32)ᵉ	0.21 (4.08)ᵉ	−0.29 (−7.11)ᵉ	−0.22 (−4.59)ᵉ	[% married X₁₀] 0.35 (2.06)	.94 (.92)
14	LW Tot. exp. (Y₁)	2.29 (4.70)ᵉ	−0.16 (−8.09)ᵉ	0.27 (4.69)ᵉ	−0.24 (−5.77)ᵉ	−0.16 (−3.37)ᵉ	[% Negro X₁₁] −0.11 (−1.45)	.93 (.91)
15	LW Hos. exp. (Y₂)	1.56 (1.51)	−0.19 (−3.87)ᵉ	0.05 (0.34)	−0.08 (−0.41)	−0.07 (−0.51)	[Ed. X₇] −2.26 (−1.44)	.77 (.69)
16	LW Med. exp. (Y₃)	2.37 (6.54)ᵉ	−0.13 (−7.71)ᵉ	0.36 (6.87)ᵉ	−0.48 (−7.15)ᵉ	−0.27 (−5.69)ᵉ	1.26 (2.28)ᵈ	.97 (.96)
17	LW Dr. exp. (Y₄)	3.06 (5.02)ᵉ	−0.12 (−4.21)ᵉ	0.38 (4.35)ᵉ	−0.39 (−3.47)ᵉ	−0.26 (−3.35)ᵉ	1.59 (1.71)	.88 (.84)
18	LW Den. exp. (Y₅)	3.20 (3.41)ᵉ	−0.12 (−2.80)ᵈ	0.22 (1.67)	0.02 (0.15)	0.04 (−0.38)	0.10 (0.07)	.71 (.60)

(continued)

TABLE 6-2 (continued)

Regressions of Medical Expenses per Currently Employed Person per Year on Various Independent Variables for Twenty-four Region-Age-Sex Cells[a]

Regression No. (1)	Form of Regression[b] and Dependent Variable (2)	Regression Coefficient and Computed t Value (in Parentheses)[c]						Biased Coefficient of Determination and Unbiased Coefficient of Determination (in Parentheses) (9)
		Income (X_1) (3)	Sex (X_2) (4)	Region (X_3) (5)	Age (X_4) or Age (X_5) (6)	Age (X_6) (7)	$X_7 - X_{12}$ (8)	
							[% married X_{10}]	
19	LW Hos. exp. (Y_2)	1.28 (1.44)	−0.31 (−4.84)[e]	0.10 (0.93)	−0.42 (−5.12)[e]	−0.31 (−3.15)[e]	1.03 (2.97)[e]	.83 (.77)
20	LW Med. exp. (Y_3)	2.23 (5.34)[e]	−0.16 (−5.35)[e]	0.28 (5.79)[e]	−0.34 (−8.88)[e]	−0.20 (−4.41)[e]	0.01 (0.05)	.96 (.95)
21	LW Dr. exp. (Y_4)	2.57 (4.67)[e]	−0.25 (−6.30)[e]	0.25 (3.80)[e]	−0.28 (−5.48)[e]	−0.25 (−4.11)[e]	0.60 (2.79)[d]	.91 (.87)
22	LW Den. exp. (Y_5)	3.33 (3.60)[e]	−0.08 (−1.20)	0.24 (2.18)[d]	0.06 (0.74)	−0.01 (−0.09)	−0.28 (−0.77)	.72 (.62)
							[% Negro X_{11}]	
23	LW Hos. exp. (Y_2)	2.04 (1.81)	−0.13 (−2.97)[e]	0.14 (1.05)	−0.34 (−3.50)[e]	−0.21 (−1.83)	0.10 (0.58)	.75 (.66)
24	LW Med. exp. (Y_3)	2.08 (4.93)[e]	−0.16 (−9.89)[e]	0.31 (6.09)[e]	−0.33 (−9.27)[e]	−0.19 (−4.48)[e]	−0.07 (−1.06)	.96 (.95)
25	LW Dr. exp. (Y_4)	2.35 (4.02)[e]	−0.18 (−7.79)[e]	0.36 (5.21)[e]	−0.18 (−3.62)[e]	−0.14 (−2.38)[d]	−0.24 (−2.63)[d]	.90 (.87)
26	LW Den. exp. (Y_5)	3.22 (3.28)[e]	−0.12 (−3.20)[e]	0.21 (1.81)	0.03 (0.40)	−0.04 (−0.43)	0.01 (0.10)	.71 (.60)
							[Earn. rate X_{12}]	
27	LW Tot. exp. (Y_1)	1.20 (2.30)[d]	−0.69 (−4.50)[e]	0.28 (6.34)[e]	−0.37 (−8.22)[e]	−0.32 (−5.94)[e]	2.07 (3.58)[e]	.96 (.94)

TABLE 6-2 (concluded)

28	LW	1.20	−0.40	0.19	−0.37	−0.25	0.96	.75
	Hos. exp. (Y_2)	(0.79)	(−0.89)	(1.50)	(−2.82)[d]	(−1.61)	(0.57)	(.66)
29	LW	1.46	−0.47	0.31	−0.41	−0.28	1.20	.97
	Med. exp. (Y_3)	(2.81)[d]	(−3.12)[e]	(7.03)[e]	(−9.08)[e]	(−5.21)[e]	(2.10)[d]	(.96)
30	LW	0.85	−0.99	0.35	−0.40	−0.40	3.15	.94
	Dr. exp. (Y_4)	(1.38)	(−5.43)[e]	(6.74)[e]	(−7.39)[e]	(−6.13)[e]	(4.60)[e]	(.92)
31	LW	2.39	−0.45	0.24	−0.03	−0.12	1.24	.72
	Den. exp. (Y_5)	(1.85)	(−1.20)	(2.22)[d]	(−0.31)	(−0.93)	(0.87)	(.62)

[a] For detailed definitions of the variables employed in the regressions, see Section 2.

[b] Natural unweighted, NU_W; natural weighted, NW; logarithmic unweighted, LU_W; logarithmic weighted, LW. The weights are obtained from the following:

Region	Age	Sex	No. of Persons	Region	Age	Sex	No. of Persons
NE	17–44	M	6,338	S	17–44	M	7,103
NE	45–64	M	3,980	S	45–64	M	3,820
NE	65—	M	525	S	65—	M	495
NE	17–44	F	3,031	S	17–44	F	3,460
NE	45–64	F	2,036	S	45–64	F	1,833
NE	65—	F	190	S	65—	F	181
NC	17–44	M	7,372	W	17–44	M	3,977
NC	45–64	M	4,236	W	45–64	M	2,205
NC	65—	M	589	W	65—	M	300
NC	17–44	F	3,181	W	17–44	F	1,800
NC	45–64	F	1,939	W	45–64	F	1,062
NC	65—	F	248	W	65—	F	102

[c] The estimated income elasticities at points of means for the natural regressions are 1.44 (regression 1) and 1.83 (regression 2).

[d] Statistically significant at the .05 level on a one-tail test for the earnings rate (X_{12}) and on a two-tail test for all other variables.

[e] Statistically significant at the .01 level on a one-tail test for the earnings rate (X_{12}) and on a two-tail test for all other variables.

found to be insignificant, and it is wisest to ignore them. The computed t value for the education variable (X_7) is more respectable but is statistically insignificant. However, in view of the wide interest in the role of this variable, it is worth noting that its sign is positive, which might be interpreted to mean that education leads individuals to take better care of their health. The coefficient of the percentage Negro (X_{11}) is negative, which might mean that, other things being equal, Negroes are healthier than whites and therefore require less medical care, but is more likely to mean that cultural and other factors result in Negroes receiving less medical care for a given problem. However, these speculations should not be emphasized, since the coefficient of X_{11} is not statistically significant. Finally, the coefficient of the marital status variable (X_{10}) is positive and is in the range of statistical significance. In order to obtain further information on the role of the last three independent variables, they were included in regressions for each of the four types of medical expense, with the results shown in regressions 15–26.

The results for the education variable (regressions 15–18) are quite interesting: the coefficient of X_7 is negative for hospital expenses, positive for medicine and physician expense, and positive but of negligible magnitude for dentist expense. A possible interpretation is that education results in emphasis being placed on preventive care, which leads to relatively low hospital and dentist expense and relatively high medicine and physician expense.[13]

The coefficient of the marital status variable is found to be positive and statistically significant for hospital and physician expense, positive but insignificant for medicine expense, and negative but insignificant for dentist expense (regressions 19–22). These results probably mean that the positive correlation between X_{10} and total expenses is a reflection of the fact that being married with a spouse present is associated with child-bearing expenses for females; child-bearing raises hospital and physician expenses but does not greatly affect dentist and medicine expenses.

It is found that the inverse relationship between the percentage Negro and total expenses is derived from a strong negative relationship for physician expense and a somewhat weaker negative effect on medicine expense (regressions 24 and 25). The basis for the observed

---

[13] Caution is justified here, as the computed t values of the education variable are not very large, and there is evidence of harmful multicollinearity in regression 15.

differences in the results for the various components is not apparent to the present writer.[14]

To the extent that analysts have been willing to take a position on this issue, they have tended to interpret positive relationships between income and medical expenses to mean that higher income permits individuals and groups to receive the benefits flowing from more and better medical care. At the same time, policy-related judgments concerning the equity of the current distribution of medical services are in part based upon the magnitude of the income elasticity. However, aside from the problems that arise in using expenses as a measure of the amount of medical care, such interpretations and judgments are spurious to the extent that (1) activities raising money incomes simultaneously depress health status and consequently increase the demand for medical services, and (2) individuals or groups with higher income use less patient-time-intensive (more medical-goods-and-services-intensive) methods of dealing with their medical problems.

Both of these conditions that give rise to upward-biased income elasticities might occur because of a positive correlation between income and the earnings rate.[15] A higher earnings rate may reduce health status while raising income by inducing individuals to "work harder," to go to work instead of staying at home when they are ill, to take more sedentary jobs, or to take more dangerous jobs. Further, it seems reasonable to believe that an increase in the earnings rate, and hence in income, will lead patients or their physicians to substitute medical goods and services for the patient's time in dealing with a given medical problem. In recognition of these possible sources of biased income elasticities, the earnings rate (X_{12}) is included in regression 27. It is found that the coefficient of the earnings rate has the expected positive sign and is statistically significant, while its inclusion lowers the income elasticity of total expenses from 2.5 (regression 5) to 1.2 and raises the adjusted coefficient of determination from 0.90 to 0.94.

In interpreting the results of the above regression it should be noted

[14] Charlotte Muller suggests that these differences may be explained by the fact that in the Negro subculture (and in other subcultures of poverty) there exists a tendency to substitute medicine for the services of physicians (self-medication) and to substitute home remedies for market purchase of medicines.

[15] Actually, the bias could be downward if (1) an increase in the volume of medical services needed to produce a given level of health resulted in a *decline* in medical expenditures (i.e., the price elasticity of demand for health was numerically greater than 1), and (2) health were relatively time-intensive and substitution in consumption outweighed substitution in production. These possibilites were called to my attention by Michael Grossman.

that the correlation coefficient between the earnings rate and sex variables is in the range of 0.9.[16] Intercorrelations of this magnitude often produce highly unstable parameter estimates. A check on the stability of the conclusions suggested by regression 27 is provided by regressions 28–31, which are for the separate components of medical expense. Although multicollinearity problems are evident in each of the regressions, the results are consistent with expectations: in every case the coefficient of the earnings rate is positive, and its inclusion in the regression causes a perceptible decline in the estimated income elasticity. The explanatory value of the earnings rate is greatest for physician expense (the adjusted coefficient of determination rises from 0.82 to 0.92) and weakest for hospital and dentist expense (virtually no change occurs in the adjusted coefficient of determination). The statistically insignificant result for dentist expense seems reasonable, since it is unlikely that higher earnings rates lead individuals to substitute money income for dental health or to use higher ratios of dental services to their own time in the production of dental health. A factor which may help to explain the exceptional showing of the earnings rate for physician expense is that in the absence of information about income doctors may discriminate in their charges on the basis of occupation, which is more highly correlated with the earnings rate than with income.

With the inclusion of the earnings rate in the regressions, the legitimacy of interpreting the estimated coefficients of income as "income elasticities" is increased. Using expected values, it is found that the elasticity for medical care as a whole is 1.2, while the elasticities for its components range from a low of 0.85 for physician expense to a high of 2.4 or 3.2[17] for dentist expense.[18]

These results demonstrate that, even when proper account is taken of the earnings rate, command over goods and services as measured by family income exerts a strong positive influence upon the amount of medical care received by individuals.[19]

[16] The correlation between the income and sex variables is only .05, while that between the earnings rate and income is .41.

[17] The latter value results when the statistically insignificant earnings rate is dropped from the regression.

[18] Medical care is produced by the market goods analyzed above together with the *patient's time*. The best available measure of the latter input is days lost from work due to illness or injury per currently employed person (Y_6), which in Section 4 is found to have an income elasticity of about 2—i.e., intermediate between medicine and dentist expense.

[19] The reader is reminded that since some free care is available to persons with very low incomes, the income elasticities in the text, which apply to the

4. REGRESSION ANALYSIS OF WORK-LOSS RATES

The primary objective of this section is to obtain information on the question of whether the work-loss rate due to illness or injury is a worthwhile addition to the currently scant stock of quantitative health measures. This purpose is accomplished by testing two hypotheses suggesting that variations in the work-loss rate reflect differences in economic variables (health status remaining constant) rather than in the objective state of health. The primary hypothesis is that the higher the earnings rate in a region-age-sex cell, the lower its rate of work loss. The secondary hypothesis is that the higher the adjusted mean total family income in a cell, the higher its work-loss rate.

The prediction concerning the earnings rate flows from both consumption and production considerations. The consumption argument runs as follows: (1) It is more pleasant to recover from an illness while resting at home than while working; (2) the earnings rate can be considered the price of the consumption good "recovery at home" or "rest"; (3) the "law of demand" predicts an inverse relationship between price and quantity. The production argument is based upon the belief that individuals with higher earnings rates (or their physicians) substitute medical goods and services for their own time in dealing with a given medical problem. Since the patient's time input is, at least in part, reflected in the work-loss rate, the above substitution results in a negative correlation between the earnings rate and the work-loss rate.

The predicted relationship between family income and the work-loss rate rests upon a consumption argument and a mixed consumption-production argument. Stated briefly, the consumption argument is that "recovery at home" or "rest" is a superior consumption good. The mixed argument is based on the assumption that health or "recovery" is a superior consumption good produced according to a production function which is homogeneous of degree one (or of any other form which excludes the possibility of "inferior" factors of production). If these assumptions hold, an increase in family income would increase the demand for health, and hence the demand for all the relevant factors of production, including the patient's own time. An increase in the patient's time input would be reflected in an increased work-loss rate.

---

relatively affluent, currently employed segment of the population, overestimate to an unknown degree the differential benefits received by the more affluent members of our society.

In order to avoid biasing the results and to increase their reliability, dummy variables representing region, age, and sex were included in the regressions shown in Table 6-3.

Negative regression coefficients for the earnings rate and positive ones for family income[20] are observed in three of the four forms utilized in regressions 1–4. In the fourth case (regression 3) the signs of family income, the earnings rate, and the sex variable (positive in the other three cases) are reversed. While none of the computed *t* values are impressive, the strongest results are obtained in regression 2, in which the positive coefficient of income is statistically significant while the negative one for the earnings rate is insignificant but respectable.

It is well known that high intercorrelations between independent variables often result in unstable parameter estimates and small computed *t* values. In the present analysis the previously noted deviant results for regression 3 and generally small computed *t* values may be symptoms of harmful multicollinearity (primarily) between the earnings rate and sex variables whose coefficient of correlation is in the range of 0.9. One method for dealing with this type of problem is to narrow the scope of the model by removing the less theoretically interesting variable, which in this case is the dummy for sex. This is done in regressions 5 and 6 for the weighted forms, which earlier yielded higher multiple correlation coefficients than the unweighted forms. It is found that the coefficients of family income and the earnings rate maintain the predicted signs and, especially in the case of the LW form, are statistically significant. The results are not greatly affected by the use of the less restrictive age variables X_5 and X_6 (see regression 7).

Of course, the danger inherent in the above precedure is that the price of avoiding harmful multicollinearity may be biased parameter estimates. Little can be done to deal with this possibility beyond running separate regressions for the twelve observations on each sex. This is done in regressions 8 and 9, which exclude the family income and region variables because they are now highly correlated with the earnings rate.[21] The results are ambiguous: while the coefficient of the male

[20] It is worth noting that the simple correlations between family income and work-loss days are small and negative.

[21] Taking all twenty-four observations together, the simple correlations between the earnings rate and the family income and regional variables are 0.41 and −0.31, respectively, while for males the corresponding values are 0.97 and −0.83 and for females, 0.89 and −0.79. The correlation between the earnings rate and age is .06 for all the observations, .21 for males, and close to 0 for females.

earnings rate is negative and statistically significant, the coefficient for females is positive and unreliable.

Obviously, the results are far from conclusive, but in my opinion they lend some support to the economic arguments presented above. The observed signs of the income and earnings rate variables, together with their relatively high partial correlation coefficients, suggest that differences in work-loss days may be unreliable measures of health status.[22] To the extent that the magnitudes of the regression coefficients can be taken seriously, it appears that the elasticity of the work-loss rate with respect to family income is surprisingly high, while that with respect to the earnings rate is low.

Turning to the other independent variables, it is found that, other things being equal, work-loss rates are higher for males, Southerners, and older persons than for females, non-Southerners, and younger persons. Like the findings for medical expenses (see Section 3), the resu.ts are consistent with the view that non-Southerners and younger persons enjoy better health than Southerners and older persons. The generally positive signs for sex are subject to a variety of interpretations, including the notion that females enjoy better health than males.

5. SUMMARY OF MAJOR FINDINGS

The empirical analysis in Section 3 reveals an income elasticity of demand of 1.2 for medical care as a whole, while the elasticities for its

[22] There are alternative, but in my opinion less plausible, interpretations according to which the empirical results are consistent with the view that the work-loss rate is a pure measure of health. First, the earnings rate might be negatively correlated with the work-loss rate because the former is an "efficiency variable"; that is, market skills might be positively correlated with skill in the production of health. Second, even after adjusting for differences in the earnings rate it might be the case that groups with higher incomes have poorer health.

A crude check of the alternative explanations presented above were obtained by running LW regressions utilizing a less ambiguous measure of health, the mortality rate, Y_M, as the dependent variable. (The mortality data utilized include deaths of persons who were not employed during the relevant period; the data were taken from the 1962 and 1963 volumes of *Vital Statistics of the United States,* from National Center for Health Statistics, *Health Insurance Coverage, United States: July 1962–June 1963,* Table 13, and from the *1960 Census of Population,* vol. 1, Pt. 1, Table 52.) The regressions offered little if any support for the alternative interpretations: (1) When the sex variable is included, the coefficient of income is positive but far from statistical significance, while the coefficient of the earnings rate is positive and insignificant; (2) when sex is dropped from the regression in order to avoid multicollinearity problems, the coefficient of income becomes *negative* and insignificant, while the coefficient of the earnings rate is positive and highly significant.

TABLE 6-3

Regressions of Days Lost from Work due to Illness or Injury per Currently Employed Person per Year (Y_6) on Various Independent Variables[a]

Regression No. (1)	Form of Regression[b] and Number of Observations (2)	Regression Coefficient and Partial Correlation Coefficient (Computed t Value in Parentheses)						Biased Coefficient of Determination and Unbiased Coefficient of Determination (in Parentheses) (9)
		Income[c] (X_1) (3)	Sex (X_2) (4)	Region (X_3) (5)	Age (X_4) or Age (X_5) (6)	Age (X_6) (7)	Earnings Rate[c] (X_7) (8)	
1	NU_w 24	0.001 0.22 (0.94)	3.55 0.26 (1.14)	2.07 0.31 (1.39)	1.42 0.53 (2.65)[d]		-0.05 -0.21 (-0.90)	.52 (.38)
2	NW 24	0.002 0.43 (2.04)[d]	3.27 0.26 (1.13)	3.23 0.56 (2.85)[d]	1.85 0.67 (3.88)[e]		-0.08 -0.32 (-1.44)	.74 (.67)
3	LU_w 24	-0.05 -0.01 (-0.06)	-0.21 -0.23 (-1.02)	0.15 0.38 (1.73)	0.13 0.67 (3.86)[e]		0.83 0.25 (1.11)	.54 (.41)
4	LW 24	1.96 0.35 (1.61)	0.02 0.02 (0.10)	0.28 0.63 (3.44)[e]	0.12 0.66 (3.69)[e]		-0.42 -0.10 (-0.42)	.77 (.71)
5	NW 24	0.001 0.39 (1.85)[d]	0.52 (2.66)[d]	2.96	2.02 0.71 (4.39)[e]		-0.02 -0.40 (-1.92)[d]	.73 (.67)

(continued)

TABLE 6-3 (concluded)

6	LW	1.86	0.64	0.27	0.12		−0.33	.77
	24	0.55			0.70		−0.53	(.72)
		(2.91)e	(3.64)e		(4.23)e		(−2.76)e	
7	LW	2.28	0.61	0.32	−0.28	−0.18	−0.33	.78
	24	0.53			−0.67	−0.45	−0.54	(.72)
		(2.64)e	(3.24)e		(−3.83)e	(−2.13)	(−2.76)e	
8	LW Males			0.24			−0.86	.82
	12			0.90			−0.56	(.78)
				(6.39)e			(−2.04)d	
9	LW Females			0.03			0.24	.18
	12			0.37			0.24	(−.00)
				(1.20)			(0.73)	

a For detailed definitions of the variables employed in the regressions, see Section 2.

b See Table 6-2, note b.

c The estimated income elasticities at points of means for the natural regressions are 0.79 (regression 1), 2.38 (regression 2), and 1.32 (regression 5). The corresponding values for the earnings rate are −0.66 (regression 1), −1.29 (regression 2), and −0.29 (regression 5).

d Statistically significant at the .05 level on a one-tail test for income and the earnings rate and on a two-tail test for all other variables.

e Statistically significant at the .01 level on a one-tail test for income and the earnings rate and on a two-tail test for all other variables.

components range from 0.85 for physician expense to 3.2 for dentist expense. The ordering of the income elasticities is not unreasonable, and the magnitudes suggest that family income exerts a strong influence upon the amount of medical care received by individuals. However, an important question for future research is why the income elasticities reported in the present study are so high relative to those estimated from other bodies of data. The elasticity of total expenses with respect to the earnings rate is positive and statistically significant and is not negligible in magnitude—its value is 2.1.

In Section 4 it is seen that the work-loss days due to illness or injury are usually positively related to family income and inversely related to the earnings rate, which suggests the tentative conclusion that differences in unadjusted work-loss days may be unreliable measures of variations in health status.

7

The Distribution of Earnings in Health and Other Industries

Victor R. Fuchs
Elizabeth Rand
Bonnie Garrett

The growing interest in the size distribution of earnings has been manifest in studies of labor income for the total work force or for large subaggregates, such as all nonfarm wage and salary workers.[1] The purpose of this note is to suggest that the size distribution of earnings within detailed industries may also merit attention. Such data can provide insights concerning the distribution of human capital within industries and the variation of these distributions across industries. In addition, the analysis of intraindustry distributions may help us to understand better certain problems in industrial organization and labor market behavior.

We compare the distribution of earnings of full-time year-round employed persons in twenty large industries. The health industry is

NOTE: This study has appeared in *The Journal of Human Resources,* 4, Summer 1970, pp. 382–89. A previously unpublished appendix, "A Note on the Distribution of Earnings in Health Under Alternative Forms of Organization," has been added here.

This paper is a by-product of the program of research at the National Bureau of Economic Research on the economics of health, supported by grants from the Commonwealth Fund and the U.S. Public Health Service (Grant 1 PO1 CH 00374-01).

Certain data used in this note were derived from punch cards furnished under a joint project sponsored by the U.S. Bureau of the Census and Population Council, and containing selected 1960 Census information for a 0.1 per cent sample of the population of the United States. Neither the Census Bureau nor the Population Council assumes any responsibility for the validity of any of the figures or interpretations of them published herein based on this material.

[1] This literature is reviewed by Jacob Mincer in "The Distribution of Labor Incomes: A Survey with Special Reference to the Human Capital Approach," *Journal of Economic Literature,* 8, March 1970.

found to have an extraordinary bimodal distribution. Possible explanations for this marked discontinuity are discussed and some questions
for further research are raised.

EARNINGS DISTRIBUTIONS

The basic data source is the 1/1,000 sample of the 1960 Census of
Population and Housing.[2] Because the relative importance of part-time
work varies considerably across industries, the study is limited to persons who worked at least forty weeks in 1959 and at least thirty hours
per week in the Census sample week in April 1960.[3] Employed persons,
including self-employed but excluding unpaid family workers, are classified by industry, and all industries, except agriculture and mining, with
at least 600 observations (i.e., 600,000 persons) are included in the
study.

Frequency distributions of annual earnings in 1959 are constructed
for each industry, and summary statistics on these distributions are
presented in Table 7-1. Mean earnings in the health industry are very
much like those of other industries. The standard deviation of earnings in health, however, is very high—almost double that of the median
industry. The coefficient of variation, which measures the relative variance or inequality in earnings, is higher for health than for any other
industry.[4] Because the distribution of earnings in many industries more
closely approximates the log normal than the normal, the coefficients
of variation of the logarithms of earnings are also shown. The health
industry again shows the greatest relative variation—almost double that
of the median industry.

In Table 7-2 the frequency distributions for each industry are allocated across earnings classes based on ratios to the industry means
rather than across specific dollar classes. This method allows us to compare distributions among industries irrespective of differing means.
Several features of the health distribution stand out. First, we notice
a much higher percentage of health workers at the very low end of the

[2] For a full description, see U.S. Department of Commerce, Bureau of the
Census, *U.S. Censuses of Population and Housing: 1960, 1/1,000, 1/10,000—
Two National Samples of the Population of the United States, Description and
Technical Documentation,* Washington, D.C.

[3] Data on hours per week in 1959 are not available.

[4] Some of the inequality is the result of positive correlation between annual
earnings and annual hours, but several rough calculations indicate that adjustment for hours of work would not alter the basic picture. The coefficient of
variation for health earnings roughly adjusted for annual hours is 1.07.

TABLE 7-1

Summary Measures of Annual Earnings of Full-Time Year-Round
Employed Persons, Twenty Large Industries, 1959

Industry	Number of Observations	Mean	Standard Deviation	Coefficient of Variation	Coefficient of Variation of Logs
Health	1,724	$5,709	$7,522	1.318	.121
Apparel	698	4,247	5,190	1.222	.096
Finance and insurance	1,902	6,200	5,853	.944	.078
Retail trade	5,866	4,772	4,277	.896	.106
Wholesale trade	1,691	6,602	5,710	.865	.082
Food	1,364	5,534	4,241	.766	.075
Textiles	692	3,837	2,841	.740	.067
Construction	2,637	5,953	4,201	.706	.077
Machinery (except electrical)	1,117	6,534	4,455	.682	.064
Printing and publishing	715	6,114	4,148	.678	.081
Electrical machinery	1,168	5,918	3,951	.668	.066
Chemicals	697	6,496	4,308	.663	.064
Transportation	2,245	5,848	3,646	.623	.068
Fabricated metals	1,372	5,680	3,425	.603	.061
Education	1,692	5,160	3,004	.582	.087
Primary metals	807	6,198	3,601	.581	.060
Communication	681	5,477	2,989	.546	.059
Utilities	803	5,525	2,615	.473	.057
Public administration (except postal)	2,118	5,459	2,550	.467	.062
Transportation equipment	1,530	6,191	2,824	.456	.049
Median	1,368	5,778	4,050	.673	.068

Note: Industry means and standard deviations are calculated using the midpoints
of each class and $40,000 for the open-ended class $25,000 and over.

distribution. Second, we note that there are very few persons in the
health industry with earnings between the mean and twice the mean.
Finally, we note that the percentage earning more than twice the mean
is much higher than in any other industry.

By selecting the median percentage distribution among the twenty
industries in each relative earnings class, we have created a "typical"
industry distribution. Comparison of the health distribution with this
"typical" distribution indicates that the greatest discrepancy is in the
range from the mean to 50 per cent above the mean; in the median

TABLE 7-2

Percentage Frequency Distributions of Earnings Relative to the Mean and Cumulative Deviations from the Median, Twenty Large Industries, 1959

Industry	Ratios to the Mean[a]									Cumulative Absolute Deviation (% Point)
	0–.25	.26–.50	.51–.75	.76–1.00	1.01–1.25	1.26–1.50	1.51–1.75	1.76–2.00	Over 2.00	
Health	9.4%	25.8%	27.7%	15.4%	5.2%	2.5%	1.7%	1.0%	11.6%	71.0
Apparel	2.2	20.7	35.1	17.4	7.3	3.8	2.9	2.1	8.4	54.9
Finance and insurance	2.6	18.0	30.0	19.2	11.1	6.5	3.7	1.5	7.4	38.0
Retail trade	6.1	17.0	21.5	18.2	13.9	8.1	4.4	2.6	8.1	33.3
Wholesale trade	3.0	15.6	25.9	23.3	12.3	5.8	4.7	3.0	6.5	26.1
Transportation equipment	0.9	4.3	19.6	35.2	22.0	9.4	4.0	2.3	2.3	24.4
Communication	0.8	6.9	29.2	24.6	14.4	11.8	5.6	2.5	4.0	19.8
Utilities	1.7	6.8	19.6	26.4	24.6	12.8	4.1	2.2	1.8	19.6
Education	4.9	9.9	18.1	23.2	19.2	11.6	5.9	2.4	4.9	19.1

(continued)

TABLE 7-2 (concluded)

Textiles	0.8	5.5	33.0	26.2	14.7	8.4	4.1	2.5	4.7	18.5
Transportation	2.1	7.0	19.6	33.0	19.2	10.0	4.3	1.8	3.1	16.3
Primary metals	1.0	6.1	22.1	34.2	19.0	7.8	4.7	1.1	4.0	15.8
Printing and publishing	1.7	12.2	23.2	20.6	20.1	10.2	5.3	1.6	5.0	15.3
Construction	3.1	11.5	22.1	24.0	16.4	11.6	4.5	2.0	4.7	15.4
Public administration (except postal)	1.0	6.2	21.5	30.4	20.4	9.3	4.7	2.3	4.1	12.3
Machinery (except electrical)	1.2	7.8	25.8	30.4	16.9	7.8	3.9	1.8	4.5	11.7
Food	2.8	11.3	20.2	27.7	19.8	8.4	3.6	1.9	4.2	11.5
Fabricated metals	1.2	6.1	24.2	29.8	20.2	8.4	4.3	2.4	3.4	10.8
Chemicals	0.9	8.5	23.1	30.5	19.0	7.8	4.0	2.6	3.6	8.2
Electrical machinery	1.5	7.9	26.8	25.7	17.6	9.6	3.9	2.1	4.8	7.5
Median[b]	1.7	8.5	24.0	26.8	18.9	8.7	4.3	2.3	4.8	17.4

[a] The classes for the frequency distributions are expressed in terms of ratios to the mean earnings for each industry. Thus, the dollar values of each class vary among industries.

[b] This distribution is referred to as the "typical" industry. The median for each class is adjusted so that the sum across classes equals 100.0.

industry about 27.6 per cent of workers fall in that range, but in health only 7.7 per cent do so. The mean earnings in health are now about $10,000, and it is not likely that any drastic change in distribution occurred during the past decade. Therefore, the current shortage is of workers whose education, experience, etc., justifies earnings of from $10,000 to $15,000 per year. These are the persons who in other industries take on middle professional and supervisory functions, freeing the more skilled so that they can concentrate on the more important and demanding tasks.[5] The data also suggest that a smaller, but signifi-cant, shortage exists in the range from one and one-half times the mean to twice the mean, i.e., in current terms, from $15,000 to $20,000 per annum. This shortage is shown graphically in Chart 7-1, where the health industry distribution is compared with that of the median or "typical" industry.

The last column in Table 7-2 presents a measure of the extent to

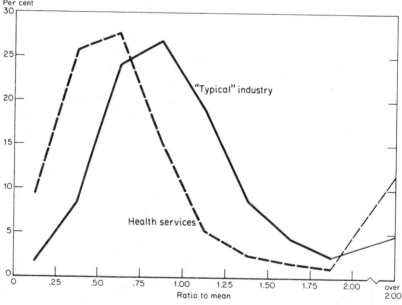

CHART 7-1

Percentage Frequency Distributions of Earnings Relative to the Mean, Health Services, and the "Typical" Industry, 1959

[5] In most industries many of these middle level workers started at lower levels and worked their way up. In the health industry, the occupational "ladders" are very limited.

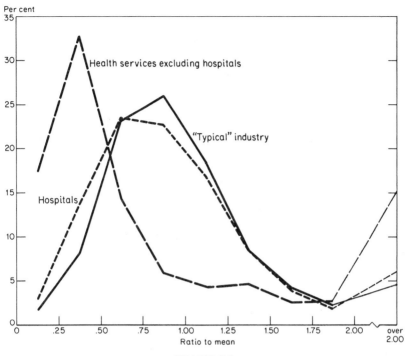

Per cent

Ratio to mean

CHART 7-2

Percentage Frequency Distributions of Earnings Relative to the Mean, Hospitals,
Health Services Excluding Hospitals, and the "Typical" Industry, 1959

which each industry's distribution departs from that of the "typical"
industry. It is the sum across the nine relative earnings classes of the
absolute deviation, in percentage points, of the given industry's frequencies from the "typical" industry's frequencies. The health industry distribution departs most from that of the "typical" industry, with a
cumulative deviation of 71.0 percentage points. The electrical machin-
ery industry has roughly one-tenth as much cumulative deviation, and
all industries except two have less than half as much deviation as does
health. Further calculations for the health industry show that its
unusual distribution of earnings is found in the four regions of the
country and in smaller cities and rural areas as well as in the large
Standard Metropolitan Statistical Areas (see Table 7-3).

When the health industry is disaggregated into "hospital" and
"medical and other health services except hospitals," we find that the
distribution of earnings in the former closely resembles that of the

TABLE 7-3

Summary Measures of Earnings Distributions in Health, by Region and City Size, 1959

	Number of Observations	Mean	Standard Deviation	Coefficient of Variation	Coefficient of Variation of Logs	Cumulative Absolute Deviation[a]
Health total	1724	$5709	$7522	1.318	.121	70.4
Region						
Northeast	501	6333	8505	1.343	.102	84.7
North Central	487	5486	7223	1.316	.102	66.8
South	464	4767	6861	1.439	.113	63.7
West	272	6566	8205	1.250	.100	74.3
City size						
SMSA's ≥ 1 million	682	6734	8669	1.287	.103	79.3
SMSA's < 1 million	521	5213	7026	1.348	.103	62.0
Outside SMSA's	521	4865	6847	1.408	.107	68.2

[a] Percentage point deviations measured from "typical" industry as defined in Table 7-2.

TABLE 7-4

Summary Measures of Earnings Distributions, Health and Other Professional Service Industries, 1959

	Number of Observations	Mean	Standard Deviation	Coefficient of Variation	Coefficient of Variation of Logs	Cumulative Absolute Deviation[a]
Hospitals	1,103	$ 3,816	$ 3,877	1.016	.085	15.5
Health, excluding hospitals	621	9,072	10,956	1.208	.121	101.5
Legal services	202	10,853	10,998	1.013	.102	73.8
Accounting services	130	7,735	7,055	.912	.082	35.4
Engineering services	148	8,079	6,588	.815	.076	26.1

[a] Percentage point deviations measured from "typical" industry as defined in Table 7-2.

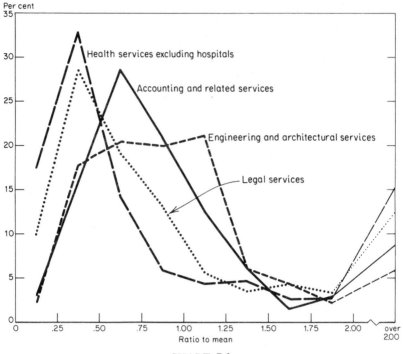

CHART 7-3

Percentage Frequency Distributions of Earnings Relative to the Mean, Four
Professional Service Industries, 1959

"typical" industry, but that the latter distribution departs even more
markedly from the "typical" than the one for health as a whole
(see Table 7-4 and Chart 7-2). This table also shows that "health excluding hospitals" departs more markedly than do the distributions for
the three other major professional service industries: legal, accounting,
and engineering (see Chart 7-3).

DISCUSSION

Several questions arise concerning the methodology and data reported
above. Are earnings a good proxy for human capital? Would distributions based on education, age, occupation, or other characteristics
reveal similar patterns? What explains the variation across industries in
the distribution of human capital? Is the distribution in health the result
of physicians' desire to prevent the emergence of any close substitutes
for their services, or is it dictated by the technology of medical care?

Is the more normal distribution observed for accounting and engineering attributable to the use of certification in those professions rather than the more restrictive licensure that prevails in law and medicine? Would the emergence of a more normal distribution of manpower in the health industry help relieve the "doctor shortage"?[6] It is hoped that this note may stimulate further research on these and related questions.

APPENDIX A:

A NOTE ON THE DISTRIBUTION OF EARNINGS IN HEALTH UNDER ALTERNATIVE FORMS OF ORGANIZATION

This note reports on a comparison between the distribution of earnings in the health industry as a whole and a single, large, prepaid group practice plan that provides comprehensive in-hospital and am-

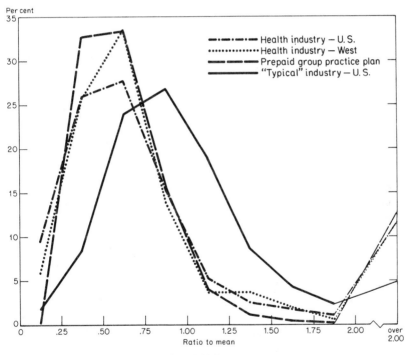

CHART 7-A-1

Percentage Frequency Distributions of Earnings Relative to the Mean, the Health Industry, the "Typical" Industry, and Prepaid Group Practice

[6] See Rashi Fein, *The Doctor Shortage: An Economic Diagnosis,* Washington, D.C., The Brookings Institution, 1967.

TABLE 7–A–1

Earnings Distributions in Prepaid Group Practice, the Health Industry,
and the "Typical" Industry

	Prepaid Group Practice Plan 1968	Health Industry U.S. 1959	Health Industry West 1959	"Typical" Industry U.S. 1959
Mean ($)	9,535	5,709	6,566	5,778
Standard deviation ($)	10,093	7,522	8,205	4,050
Coefficient of variation (%)	105.8	131.8	125.0	67.3
Frequency distributions (%) (ratios to the mean)				
0–0.25	0.1	9.4	5.8	1.7
0.26–0.50	33.7	25.8	25.7	8.5
0.51–0.75	32.9	27.7	33.4	24.0
0.76–1.00	15.2	15.1	13.8	26.8
1.01–1.25	3.8	5.2	3.7	18.9
1.26–1.50	1.0	2.5	3.7	8.7
1.51–1.75	.4	1.7	1.9	4.3
1.76–2.00	.1	1.0	0.5	2.3
Over 2.00	12.8	11.6	11.6	4.8

bulatory care. Many advocates of prepaid group practice have suggested that one of the advantages of this type of organization is the opportunity it affords for restructuring the inputs of personnel at different levels of skill and responsibility.[7] In particular, it is thought that a prepaid plan offering comprehensive outpatient as well as hospital care could economize in the use of physicians and make more use of technicians and other middle-level personnel.

Table 7–A–1 compares the prepaid group practice plan with the U.S. health industry and the "typical" U.S. industry.[8] A comparison with the health industry in the West, the region in which the prepaid group practice plan under discussion is located, is also presented. Chart 7–A–1 shows the percentage frequency distributions in graphical form.

We see that the distribution of earnings in the prepaid group practice plan is similar to that for the health industry in the United States

[7] Fein, *The Doctor Shortage*, 1967; also, A. A. Boan, *Group Practice*, Ottawa, Royal Commission on Health Service, Queen's Printer, 1966.

[8] The "typical" industry is based on the median of twenty large industries in the United States.

as a whole and in the West. The coefficient of variation, which measures the relative inequality of earnings, is slightly smaller for the plan, but the shortage of workers earning more than the mean but less than twice the mean is even more pronounced than in the health industry as a whole.

There are, to be sure, significant differences in the series being compared. The three general series refer to 1959 and are based on unverified responses to household interviews, and the mean and standard deviations are calculated using frequency distribution midpoints. The plan data refer to 1968 and use the mean (since it is known) rather than the estimated midpoint of the open-ended class.

These differences may bias the distributions, but it seems unlikely that they could account for the striking similarity in all the health series and the sharp differences between the health series and other industries. The introduction of a different form of financing and delivery of health care has apparently not resulted in a significantly different mix of personnel. To the extent that the prepaid group practice plan is more efficient, it probably takes the form of a saving in all types of personnel, not in the substitution of middle-level professionals for the more expensive physicians.

PART III

THE PRODUCTION OF HEALTH

8

The Production of Health, an Exploratory Study

Richard Auster
Irving Leveson
Deborah Sarachek

INTRODUCTION: THE PROBLEM

The medical industry is one of the most important and one of the fastest-growing industries in the United States. Moreover, it is an industry in which government plays a large and increasing role.[1] Government activities now encompass the sponsorship or undertaking of most medical research, the financing of medical care and hospital construction, the regulation of the supply of personnel and the practice of medicine, and the financing of medical education. Government decisions

NOTE: This paper has been reprinted from *The Journal of Human Resources*, 4, Fall 1969, pp. 412–36.

The research was done under the auspices of the National Bureau of Economic Research "Productivity in the Service Industries" project, financed by a grant from the Ford Foundation; and the "Economics of Health Program," financed by a grant from the Commonwealth Fund; with a grant of computer time from the IBM Corporation. The authors wish to express thanks to Victor R. Fuchs for his encouragement and support as well as for his extensive comments and suggestions. Without his pioneering work, this study would not have been possible. Also appreciated is the assistance rendered in the form of comments and criticism by Gary Becker, Philip Enterline, Michael Grossman, Reuben Gronau, Herbert Klarman, Sidney Leveson, John Meyer, Robert Michael, Jacob Mincer, David O'Neill, Melvin Reder, and Morris Silver. Finally, thanks are due to Robin Ringler, Ira Silver, Lorraine Wolch, and, especially, Henrietta Lichtenbaum for research assistance.

All appendixes referred to and additional tables are available from the authors upon request.

[1] In recent years almost one-third of national health expenditure has been made by government. Total medical care spending is now running at an annual rate in excess of $50 billion. While employment in the United States has grown at a rate of 1.2 per cent per year since 1929, employment in the health industry has grown at 3.5 per cent.

affect the way in which resources are allocated between health and other goals, between medical services and other determinants of health, and among the various types of medical services. (The term "medical" services is used here to include public health activities.) If such allocation decisions are to be optimal it is necessary to know both the costs of and returns to each possible use. While in similar fields, such as education, information on returns has become increasingly available, in the health field work has largely centered on costs alone.

Recently some attempts have been made to evaluate the economic benefits of improvements in health.[2] However, as yet no one has answered in a satisfactory way the very basic question, "What is the contribution of medical services as opposed to environmental factors to changes in the health of the population?" (The term "environmental factors" is used here simply to refer to all factors other than medical and health services.) Certainly, more studies of the effects of specific therapeutic techniques on health and of the role of the factors of production in individual health programs are needed.[3] However, for broad policy questions, there is also a need for the measurement of the over-all effect of "medical services" on health and of the contribution of each of the factors of production which combine to produce "medical services."

Past studies of the factors influencing health have commonly dealt with a few variables at a time. Information on the effectiveness of medical services in improving health has typically been derived from the relatively few deliberate or "natural" experiments whose results were such as to make the impact of medical care easily discernible. The situations that were the subject of these experiments have been limited to a relatively small part of the health spectrum; most of them were in areas where medical accomplishments have been atypically great. Moreover, for a growing range of problems the importance of environmental conditions makes it impossible to determine adequately the impact of medical services on health solely in experimental circum-

---

[2] For example, see Selma J. Mushkin, "Health as an Investment," *Journal of Political Economy,* supplement, October 1962, pp. 129–57; Burton A. Weisbrod, *Economics of Public Health,* Philadelphia, University of Pennsylvania Press, 1961; Victor R. Fuchs, "Some Economic Aspects of Mortality in the United States," National Bureau of Economic Research, July 1965, mimeo.; Mary Lou Larmore, "An Inquiry into an Econometric Production Function for Health in the United States," Ph.D. dissertation, Northwestern University, August 1967.

[3] For a summary of some of these studies, see the first essay in this volume by Victor R. Fuchs.

stances. For these problems, a broad attempt to separate environmental effects from the impact of medical care on health is desirable, both as a policy guide and as an indicator of directions for further study. The influence of socioeconomic factors on health has frequently been considered apart from studies of the impact of medical care. In order to properly determine the role of medical care and other forces, both are best considered together.

The following sections describe variants of an econometric model designed to determine the causes of geographic variation in health, estimate the coefficients of the model, and consider some of their implications.

THE MODEL

Some of the most difficult problems in medical economics revolve around the definition and measurement of the output of the medical and health services industry. If we define output according to the services provided, our definition would imply such measures as physicians' visits and patient days in hospitals. Under such a definition, productivity analysis would be concerned with the production of medical services themselves. If, however, the production process is viewed as one that changes the health status of the population, medical services must be considered as an intermediate product in the "production" of health.[4] Because of our concern with the impact of medical services on health we take the latter approach. This deviates from the usual practice of defining output as a good or service. We define output as the result derived from the use of that good or service, because we are primarily interested in finding ways to improve health.[5] Moreover, because of consumer ignorance about the impact of medical services on health, the possibility that medical services are not competitively priced, and a conceivable divergence between private and social benefits we are not willing to assume that the optimum quantity of medical care is already being provided. Instead, we would like to

[4] See Victor R. Fuchs's first essay in this volume, pp. 3–38. See also Kenneth E. Boulding, "The Concept of Need for Health Services," *Milbank Memorial Fund Quarterly,* 44, October 1966, pp. 202–21.

[5] Defining the output of the medical industry by medical outcomes is similar to Lancaster's focus on attributes of goods and services and Becker's on characteristics. See Kelvin Lancaster, "A New Approach to Consumer Theory," *Journal of Political Economy,* 74, April 1966, and Gary S. Becker, "A Theory of the Allocation of Time," *Economic Journal,* 75, September 1965.

determine the benefits of medical care and compare them with costs, to arrive at judgments as to whether additional expenditures are warranted.

Given the amount of medical services that a group of individuals consumes and some socioeconomic variables, it should be possible to predict what the health of the group will be. We assume that genetic factors are either reasonably constant across states, or do not vary systematically with our independent variables, and that consequently the other variables are not influenced by genetic effects on health. Thus, we hypothesize that health will be a function of the amount of medical services (M) consumed in that state and of the following environmental variables.[6]

Per cent nonwhite (X_0). At a given level of income, education, et cetera, nonwhites may have poorer sanitation, housing, et cetera as a result of discrimination.

Income (X_1). It has been observed that higher-income people tend to consume higher-quality goods, better housing, et cetera, which may favorably affect their health. On the other hand, high incomes may permit a general style of life that is not conducive to health, particularly because the individual may be able to compensate for the adverse effects of his consumption pattern by simultaneously consuming more medical care. In addition, an increase in income may require entering those occupations which involve less exercise and/or more tension. This variable acts as a proxy for a host of factors for which we would prefer specific measures.

Education (X_2). Higher levels of education may be associated with relatively more medical care at preventive stages. In addition, the better educated may provide more care for themselves or members of their families, or simply be more willing to take the doctor's advice.

Standard Metropolitan Statistical Areas (SMSA's), per cent of population inside SMSA's (X_3). Urbanization may have adverse effects on health because of such factors as air and water pollution, congestion, et cetera.

Per cent employed in manufacturing (X_4). This index of industrialization was found to be significant by Fuchs. It may reflect patterns of work or simply general air pollution.

Alcohol consumption per capita (X_5) *and cigarette consumption per capita* (X_6). These two consumption items are included explicitly because of their special interest and our ability to measure them.

---

[6] The sources and methods used are given in Appendix A.

Per cent in white-collar occupations (X_7). This is a proxy variable for factors like stress and exercise.

Females not in the labor force (per cent of females not in the labor force, married, with husband present) (X_8). If labor force activity is more adverse to health than household activity, this variable will be positively related to health. In addition, women out of the labor force provide medical services to other members of their families. It may not be highly skilled care, but it is personal and in the right place at the right time. If there is important variation in such home production, the variable will also tend to have a positive relation to health.

We also add a variable indicating the effectiveness of medical care: *Medical school (a dummy variable coded 1 for states with medical schools and 0 for those without)* (X_9). It is hypothesized that the quality of medical care will be higher and the technology more advanced in hospitals associated with medical schools than in others. Also, it is assumed that medical schools disseminate information and provide continuous training to physicians in the community.

Specifically, we write the following production function for health:[7]

$$H = A_1 M^{\sigma_0} \prod_{i=1}^{9} X_i^{\sigma_i} e^{\epsilon_1} \tag{1}$$

where ϵ_1 is a random disturbance term which is assumed to be normally distributed. We intend in this formulation (Model I) to measure M by expenditures on medical care per capita (E). The price elasticity of demand for medical services appears to be very close to zero. Price variation may therefore act similarly to measurement error in an independent variable which, if uncorrelated with the dependent variable,

---

[7] This equation involves two further assumptions: first, that the amount of medical services produced in an area equals the amount consumed there; second, that health is a function of this year's medical services only, i.e., that the state of the group's health is not affected by the amount of medical services or environmental factors prevailing over the lifetimes of members of the group. Correlations for the various variables by state between the years 1940, 1950, and 1960 are very high, indicating that relative conditions in each state have not changed greatly over time. As a test of whether this is a source of serious bias, a migration variable was introduced into the production equation. The results (not shown) were not materially affected. Inclusion of variables for the years in question would introduce a high degree of multicollinearity into our estimates. The adverse effects of this would most likely outweigh the benefits from improved specification. The related problem of selective migration was examined by comparing the difference between deaths by state of residence and deaths by state of occurrence with residuals from early runs and found unimportant.

would bias the regression coefficient of expenditures downward. An alternative formulation will be considered later.

The primary purpose of this paper is to estimate σ_0, the elasticity of health with respect to medical services. This could be done directly by estimating equation (1) by ordinary least squares. However, to do so would result in biased estimates owing to the simultaneous nature of the problem. This can be illustrated by considering the meaning of the coefficient of physicians in an equation relating it and other variables to health. One is tempted to interpret this coefficient as a measure of the effect of doctors on health. Consider, however, that where health is poor, ceteris paribus, the demand for doctors will tend to be high. If doctors move around the country in such a way as to equalize returns to medical practice, then areas with poor health will tend to attract a greater than average number of doctors per capita. Or, to put the matter more precisely, not only does the coefficient in question measure the elasticity of health with respect to doctors, but also the elasticity of doctors with respect to health. In order to deal with the simultaneity, estimates are obtained by using two-stage least squares. This technique involves the replacement of each independent endogenous variable in equation (1) by predicted values obtained by regressing that variable on all of the exogenous variables in the model.[8] Equations for the demand for medical services, and the supplies of physicians, paramedical personnel,[9] and hospital capital[10] were specified. These equations, together with equation (1), give us the following set of exogenous variables:

X_0 Per cent nonwhite
X_1 Income
X_2 Education
X_3 Per cent of population inside SMSA's
X_4 Per cent employed in manufacturing
X_5 Alcohol consumption per capita
X_6 Cigarette consumption per capita
X_7 Per cent in white-collar occupations
X_8 Married women out of the labor force
X_9 Medical school
X_{10} Per cent of population more than sixty years old
X_{11} Birth rate

[8] See J. Johnston, *Econometric Methods,* New York, McGraw-Hill Book Co., 1963, chap. 9.

[9] All persons employed in the industry "medical and other health services," with the exception of physicians and surgeons.

[10] The derivation and estimation of these equations are contained in Appendixes C and D, and the basic data, in Appendixes F and G.

X_{12} Per cent foreign born
X_{13} Per cent of health expenditures financed by health insurance
X_{14} Per cent of health expenditures in state and local governmental short-term hospitals
X_{15} Per cent of population rural
X_{16} Per cent of population in SMSA's of 1 million or more
X_{17} Ratio of 1960 to 1950 population
X_{18} Total property income
X_{19} Labor force participation rate of females

The classification of variables as endogenous or exogenous is necessarily somewhat arbitrary and is dictated in part by the completeness of our model. Consideration of classifications implied by other models is beyond the scope of this article.

As an alternative to measuring medical services by expenditures, we can specify a production function for medical services. Specifically, we can write

$$M = A_1 D^{\alpha_1} N^{\alpha_2} K^{\alpha_3} R^{\alpha_4} G^{\alpha_5} X_9{}^{\alpha_0} e^{\epsilon_2} \qquad (2)$$

where

D = number of physicians per capita,
N = number of paramedical personnel per capita,
K = medical capital per capita,
R = prescription drug expenditures per capita,
G = per cent of practicing physicians in group practice, and
X_9 = medical school.

Note that in addition to the four input measures, two efficiency variables—group practice and medical school—are included. Many people believe that medical care produced in group practice (G) tends to have a more favorable end result because the care is more continuous and there is better exchange of information between the physicians. We expect a positive coefficient for this variable in equation (2) and a negative coefficient in equation (3) below. Substituting equation (2) into equation (1) yields

$$H = (A_1 A_2{}^{\sigma_0}) \, (D^{\alpha_1} N^{\alpha_2} K^{\alpha_3} R^{\alpha_4} G^{\alpha_5} X_9{}^{\alpha_6})^{\sigma_0} \prod_{i=1}^{4} X_i^{\sigma_i} e^{\epsilon_1 + \epsilon_2}.$$

If we then impose the restriction that $\sum_{i=1}^{4} \alpha_i = 1$, that is, that the production function of medical services exhibits constant returns to scale, we can obtain an estimate of σ_0 by summing the coefficients of D, N, K, and R; that is,

$$\sigma_0\alpha_1 + \sigma_0\alpha_2 + \sigma_0\alpha_3 + \sigma_0\alpha_4 = \sigma_0 \sum_{i=1}^{4} \alpha_i = \sigma_0 \,. \qquad (3)$$

Equation (3) together with the exogenous variables listed for Model I will be referred to as Model II; Models I and II will enable us to investigate the impact of medical services and environmental factors on health. This will be done by an analysis of interstate differences in health in 1960.[11]

MEASUREMENT OF HEALTH

The growing awareness that as the incomes of nations grow, medical services are devoted to an increasing number of problems—disability, mental illness, problems of aging, et cetera—has caused researchers to devise an ever increasing number and variety of measures to supplement the use of death rates. Among these are measures of the prevalence of chronic conditions and activity limitations, and measures of work loss and bed disability.

Measures of mortality possess a number of properties which make them suitable for health research. They are objectively measured, reasonably accurate, readily available, and universally understood. Their use in any new study has the feature of comparability with earlier work.[12] However, even within the class of mortality measures,

[11] The use of individuals rather than states as the unit of observation would present many problems because of transitory influences. For example, high-income individuals might have better health because those with poor health can work less frequently or earn lower wages. The use of states requires attention to the distribution of characteristics and resources among individuals because relationships among aggregates may depend on them. However, it reduces the importance of transitory factors. One reason for this is that health is likely to vary much less relative to variation in income across states than across individuals. Another advantage of using states is that medical knowledge probably varies less across them than over time or across countries, at least for recent years, when the death rate has changed little. Finally, with states, variations in reporting practices and in the accuracy of information, which may be serious at the individual level, tend to average out.

[12] Fuchs points out that the ranks across geographic divisions of measures of mortality and morbidity tend to be correlated in spite of inadequacies in the morbidity measures. The lowest correlations are with measures indicating the presence of chronic conditions. For example, the rank correlation of age-adjusted death rates with age-adjusted average work-loss days per person seventeen years and older is 0.65, while it is only 0.08 with the age-adjusted percentage of persons with one or more chronic conditions and some activity limitation. See "Some Economic Aspects of Mortality," Table 2.

many indices have been used in the past. These indices differ according to whether they are crude death rates or rates standardized to a common age distribution, or whether they are death rates for specific age groups or for all age groups combined. In some cases life expectancy has been used.[13]

Age- and sex-specific death rates are preferred in principle, but not enough information was available to derive measures of the amount of medical care each age or sex group receives. It did not seem reasonable to assume that the relative use of medical services per capita in each age group was the same in every state, in spite of variations in relative income, education, et cetera. The decision was made to examine age–sex-adjusted death rates.

The use of age-adjusted death rates as the measure of health for the purpose of determining the impact of medical services presumes that a constant proportion of medical services is devoted to prolonging life as opposed to reducing pain or other health-related goals. The use of an insufficiently comprehensive measure of health can lead to biased measurement of the impact of medical services on health. For example, we might understate the effect of medical care on mortality if a relatively large proportion of medical services tended to be used

[13] Different patterns of age-specific death rates can result in the same average age at death; even when they do, people may prefer one pattern over another. Average life expectancy is in principle superior to age-adjusted death rates, since it takes into account not only variation in the average age at death but also differences in patterns of age-specific death rates. Once the importance of the entire distribution of age-specific death rates is recognized, a number of other measures of aspects of health are immediately suggested. For any given average age at death, a greater or lesser dispersion of the average age at death across individuals, or other characteristics of the distribution, may be considered desirable. Persons who weigh more immediate improvements more heavily than later ones may at any given age feel better off from a reduction in age-specific death rates in age groups which they are immediately approaching than from an even larger reduction in the future, even though that larger reduction has a greater effect on average life expectancy. This suggests still another measure: a "discounted life expectancy" that gives greater weight to more immediate gains.

The difference in geographic patterns between life expectancy and age-adjusted death rates (adjusted to the U.S. age distribution by the indirect method) is small in the United States at the present time. The correlation coefficient between the two measures across states in 1960 is 0.96. The life expectancy data were supplied by Harley B. Messenger.

A number of readers have mentioned the possibility of omitting violent deaths. These are intended to be influenced by medical care, as are "natural" deaths. In any event, they are a small part of the total and their exclusion would have little effect.

for goals other than to prolong life in states using large amounts of medical care per capita. This problem is considered further in discussing the results.

THE RESULTS

Determinants of Death Rates—Model I

Initially, we attempted to determine the production relationship for whites and nonwhites combined. Table 8-1 presents Model I results for this specification, estimated by ordinary least squares. The large positive coefficient of color would imply that nonwhites experience higher death rates than whites, holding constant both the levels of socioeconomic variables and the quantity of medical care. Percentage nonwhite is correlated with many of the other variables, making it difficult to separate their effects from variation associated with color and introducing some doubt as to the accuracy of the estimated effect of the color variable itself. For example, the partial correlation between color and education, given income, is 0.44. Because differences between whites and nonwhites are great for many of the other independent variables, treating whites and nonwhites together raises the intercor-

TABLE 8-1
Production of Health, Total Population, Model I,
Ordinary Least Squares

		Linear		Log	
		Regression Coefficient	Standard Error	Regression Coefficient	Standard Error
Intercept		6.776	.783	.860	.164
Per cent nonwhite	(X_0)	.054	.008	.048	.009
Income	(X_1)	.057	.029	.023	.084
Education	(X_2)	− .152	.086	− .153	.138
Per cent in SMSA's	(X_3)	− .002	.003	− .012	.006
Per cent in manufacturing	(X_4)	.008	.007	.049	.020
Alcohol consumption per capita	(X_5)	.060	.197	.031	.046
Cigarette consumption per capita	(X_6)	− .019	.011	.141	.063
Health expenditures per capita	(E)	− .084	.007	− .084	.081
Medical school	(X_9)	− .020	.158	− .020	.011
R^2		.761		.674	

relation among these variables. Because color may interact with other variables, there is also a possibility of specification error. When whites are considered alone, correlation between education and income falls from 0.73 to 0.55 (see Table 8-2) and between education and medical care, from 0.67 to 0.47. On the basis of the above considerations, it was decided to restrict the analysis to whites.

Table 8-3 presents Model I estimates by ordinary least squares for

TABLE 8-2
Correlation Coefficients, White Population, Logarithms

	Age–Sex-adjusted Death Rate (H')	Income (X'₁)	Education (X'₂)	Per Cent in SMSA's (X'₃)	Per Cent in Manufacturing (X'₄)
Income (X')	.447				
Education (X'₂)	− .044	.551			
Per cent in SMSA's (X'₃)	.112	.265	− .112		
Per cent in manufacturing (X'₄)	.381	.278	− .195	.273	
Alcohol consumption per capita (X₅)	.378	.671	.330	.172	.021
Cigarette consumption per capita (X₆)	.478	.463	.224	.050	.116
Health expenditures per capita (E)	.166	.680	.467	.230	.061
Medical school (X₉)	.100	.085	.161	.352	.611

TABLE 8-3
Production of Health, White Population, Model I,
Ordinary Least Squares

		Linear		Log	
		Regression Coefficient	Standard Error	Regression Coefficient	Standard Error
Intercept		.957	.099	− .196	.152
Income	(X'₁)	.003	.002	.204	.076
Education	(X'₂)	− .016	.011	− .218	.112
Per cent in SMSA's	(X'₃)	− .000	.000	− .000	.005
Per cent in manufacturing	(X'₄)	.002	.001	.040	.018
Alcohol consumption per capita	(X₅)	.013	.027	− .002	.038
Cigarette consumption per capita	(X₆)	.002	.002	.102	.056
Health expenditures per capita	(E)	− .001	.001	− .065	.065
Medical school	(X₉)	− .042	.021	− .023	.010
R^2		.517		.539	

whites, in both linear and logarithmic forms. In the logarithmic form, the regression coefficients are elasticities. Variables for whites were used where possible. These are indicated by a "prime" over the variable number. It was necessary to assume that the per capita usage of medical services by whites in a state is the same as for the entire population. Fuchs experimented with the assumption that the share of medical services received by whites is the same as their share of income, and found that the regression coefficients of the modified measures of medical services differed little from the original ones. This was found for our study also.

More than 50 per cent of the variation among states in age–sex-adjusted death rates is associated with the combination of medical and environmental variables. The sign of health expenditures is negative, contrary to the positive zero order correlation. A 10 per cent increase reduces mortality by two-thirds of a per cent in the logarithmic form. Income is positively related to the death rate, while education has a negative association. This finding is not the result of intercorrelation between the two variables. The coefficient for income remains positive after the education variable is omitted. The same signs appear even in the simple correlations. Also, the use of the age-adjusted income and education measures does not change the results. Urbanization does not appear to be important when other factors are held constant, either in the form shown or when alternative measures are used. However, the index of industrialization—percentage of employment in manufacturing—is positively related to mortality. Cigarette consumption per capita exhibits a positive association with mortality, but alcohol consumption does not have a consistently positive sign.[14] The effect of per capita medical services appears to be small, but, as was indicated in the previous section, estimates of the effect of medical services on

---

[14] Alternative estimates of the coefficients of alcohol, cigarettes, and percentage in manufacturing were derived from the demand estimating equation in Appendix C. These are 0.006, 0.200, and 0.029, respectively; all three are very similar to those presented in this section. In the case of alcohol, some measure of the distribution of its use might be helpful. While we have hypothesized a positive coefficient for urbanization, it should be noted that the single most important variable explaining interstate differences in motor vehicle accident death rates is population density—with a negative sign. See Victor R. Fuchs and Irving Leveson, "Motor Accident Mortality and Compulsory Inspection of Vehicles," *Journal of the American Medical Association,* 201, August 28, 1967, pp. 657–61. Since we include accidental deaths and since population density is positively related to urbanization, urbanization may be measuring two things with opposite effects on "health," i.e., pollution and speed of cars.

the death rate by ordinary least squares are subject to simultaneous equations bias. States with medical schools tend to have lower mortality rates than those without them. A coefficient of -0.02 in the logarithmic form implies that states with medical schools, all other things being equal, have lower death rates by 4.5 per cent than states without medical schools.[15] A related variable—percentage of physicians in active practice under age thirty-five (excluding interns and residents)—was also tested. It was intended to measure the vintage of the available technology. The effects of the variable, however, disappeared when the medical school variable was introduced. Another efficiency parameter considered was hospital size, which was thought a possible reflection of quality of care. However, it did not show the expected sign, while it increased problems of multicollinearity.

Table 8-4 presents estimates for Model I using two-stage least squares (2SLS). The standard errors cannot be clearly interpreted, since when 2SLS is used, the underlying distributions are not known. They may nevertheless serve as a guide. As expected, the coefficient of per capital medical expenditures was increased (to -0.116, with a standard error of 0.082).[16] The other coefficients were essentially unchanged.

TABLE 8-4

Production of Health, White Population, Model I,
Two-Stage Least Squares, Logarithms

		Regression Coefficient	Standard Error
Intercept		$-.135$	.162
Income	(X'_1)	.212	.075
Education	(X'_2)	$-.194$	.114
Per cent in SMSA's	(X'_3)	$-.000$	.005
Per cent in manufacturing	(X'_4)	.039	.018
Alcohol consumption per capita	(X_5)	.014	.041
Cigarette consumption per capita	(X_6)	.099	.056
Health expenditure per capita[a]	(E)	$-.116$	.082
Medical school	(X_9)	$-.021$	.010
R^2		.551	

[a] Endogenous.

[15] A continuous form of this variable performed less satisfactorily. The dummy variable is still coded zero and one in logarithmic equations but is interpreted as the log of a variable coded one and ten.

[16] This probably results not only from the removal of simultaneous equation bias but also in part from the elimination of measurement error in the medical expenditures variable by the use of the instruments in the first stage.

In Table 8-5 two variables are added to the two-stage least squares equation. At this point, it should be emphasized that, with the nature of the data available, improved specification often comes at the price of a radical increase in multicollinearity. While the increase in multicollinearity from the addition of the white-collar and labor-force variables is not very destructive in this case, it would be if they were included in Model II. The proportion of workers in white-collar occupations is positively associated with death rates, while the proportion of married females with husband present and out of the labor force is negatively associated with mortality. The inclusion of these two variables appreciably increases the coefficient of determination at the same time as it reduces the estimated effect of medical care on mortality.[17]

Determinants of Death Rates—Model II

Model II disaggregates medical services into four components. It is expected that this disaggregation will raise the estimate of the effect of medical services on the death rate. In the form "medical expenditures," part of the variation results from variations in price as distinguished from quantity, the former having no relevance for the death rate. To the extent that price variation operates as a kind of random measurement error, variation in expenditures will tend to overstate the true variation in quantity and result in an understatement of the regression coefficient.[18] All Model II equations are in logarithmic form. Table 8-6

---

[17] Two hypotheses can be advanced to explain the effect of the female labor force variable. Labor market activity may be less favorable to health than non-market activity. Also, females at home may provide unmeasured medical services. The former would suggest that the relationship would hold for females; the latter that it would hold for males. In fact, the coefficient is very close to zero in regressions against the white male age-adjusted death rate, but is quite large for females. However, this cannot be clearly interpreted as support for the market activity hypothesis. In states where the death rate of males relative to females is high, relatively more females will be widowed and/or working. The female labor force variable, therefore, is in part a proxy for the ratio of the male to the female death rate which is correlated with the sex-specific death rates in such a way as tend to produce the observed result. On the other hand, relatively more women will be out of the labor force where the health of women is poor. The net effect of these two biases is not known.

[18] Even if price did not vary, the expenditure variable, which as measured here is essentially total cost, would only be an error-free measure of the quantity of medical services if the production function were homogeneous of degree one and factors of production were being combined in a cost-minimizing way. The latter, in particular, is not necessarily true in a nonprofit industry.

TABLE 8-5

Production of Health, White Population, Two-Stage Least Squares, Logarithms

		White-Collar Workers		Females Not in Labor Force		White-Collar Workers and Females Not in Labor Force	
		Regression Coefficient	Standard Error	Regression Coefficient	Standard Error	Regression Coefficient	Standard Error
Intercept		−.287	.175	.232	.251	.126	.240
Income	(X'_1)	.168	.076	.226	.074	.177	.072
Education	(X'_2)	−.243	.113	−.244	.113	−.312	.110
Per cent in SMSA's	(X'_3)	−.002	.005	.000	.005	−.003	.004
Per cent in manufacturing	(X'_4)	.048	.018	.025	.019	.034	.018
Alcohol consumption per capita	(X_5)	.014	.040	.006	.040	.004	.038
Cigarette consumption per capita	(X_6)	.099	.054	.084	.054	.080	.051
White-collar workers	(X'_7)	.145	.075			.173	.072
Females not in labor force	(X'_8)			−.233	.124	−.281	.119
Health expenditures per capita[a]	(E)	−.096	.080	−.090	.081	−.061	.077
Medical school	(X_9)	−.028	.010	−.016	.010	−.023	.010
R^2			.591		.589		.645

[a] Endogenous in two-stage least squares runs.

TABLE 8-6

Production of Health, Model II, Without Composites

		Ordinary Least Squares		Two-Stage Least Squares	
		Regression Coefficient	Standard Error	Regression Coefficient	Standard Error
Intercept		−.065	.157	.037	.251
Income	(X'_1)	.105	.079	.183	.116
Education	(X'_2)	−.161	.121	−.288	.216
Per cent in SMSA's	(X'_3)	−.001	.005	−.001	.005
Per cent in manufacturing	(X'_4)	.051	.023	.042	.040
Alcohol consumption per capita	(X_5)	−.002	.037	.013	.044
Cigarette consumption per capita	(X_6)	.094	.053	.097	.058
Drug expenditures per capita[a]	(R)	−.070	.040	−.076	.066
Physicians per capita[a]	(D)	.143	.064	.044	.111
Paramedical per capita[a]	(N)	−.190	.076	−.031	.195
Capital per capita[a] (plant assets)	(K)	−.004	.048	−.109	.141
Group practice[a]	(G)	.007	.012	.007	.021
Medical school	(X_9)	−.034	.012	−.024	.019
R^2		.639		.586	
Elasticity of the death rate with respect to medical services (σ_0)		−.121		−.172	

[a] Endogenous in two-stage least squares runs.

presents estimates of Model II by ordinary least squares and instrumental variables. Capital is measured by the value of plant assets. (The problem of capital measurement is discussed in Appendix B.) As was to be expected, the instrumental variables estimation yields a higher estimate of σ_0 than ordinary least squares; higher values for σ_0 are also obtained vis-à-vis Model I. The coefficients of the environmental variables differ little between the top models. While σ_0, the sum of the coefficients of the factors of production, is fairly constant between alternative formulations, determination of the effects of individual factors of production is hampered by the high intercorrelations among these factors. The highest degree of correlation is between paramedical personnel and capital. In an attempt to eliminate this, the two variables were combined by linearly regressing the total number of paramedical personnel on capital and combining the factors according to the estimated conversion.[19] Estimates using this "composite" are shown in Table 8-7. The elasticity of the death rate with respect to medical services is —0.134 in the two-stage least squares run, and the positive coefficient of physicians is reduced to zero. The environmental coefficients are essentially unchanged.[20] In such gross comparisons, no impact of group practice on mortality is discernible.

An attempt was made to deal more adequately with variations in the quality of physicians, in particular between general practitioners and specialists. A fixed weight composite of G.P.'s and specialists based on the national difference in their earnings was used. In addition,

TABLE 8-7

Production of Health, Model II, Composite of Capital and Paramedical Personnel

		Ordinary Least Squares		Two-Stage Least Squares	
		Regression Coefficient	Standard Error	Regression Coefficient	Standard Error
Intercept		.018	.181	— .044	.213
Income	(X'_1)	.165	.075	.183	.080
Education	(X'_2)	— .263	.108	— .231	.116
Per cent in SMSA's	(X'_3)	— .002	.005	.000	.006
Per cent in manufacturing	(X'_4)	.035	.023	.039	.029
Alcohol consumption per capita	(X_5)	— .014	.038	.008	.044
Cigarette consumption per capita	(X_6)	.108	.055	.098	.059
Drug expenditures per capita[a]	(R)	— .062	.042	— .051	.064
Physicians per capita[a]	(D)	.089	.061	.003	.090
Composite of capital and paramedical per capita[a] (plant assets)	$(K + N)$	— .124	.061	— .086	.072
Group practice[a]	(G)	.001	.012	.001	.017
Medical school	(X_9)	— .028	, .012	— .022	.015
R^2		.595		.557	
Elasticity of the death rate with respect to medical services (σ_0)		— .097		— .134	

[a] Endogenous in two-stage least squares runs.

[19] The relationship indicated fixed proportions.

[20] In an attempt to treat incomes as an endogenous variable, the endogenous form was more highly correlated with other variables and its coefficient increased.

composites of paramedical and alternative measures of capital input were considered. The use of the physicians' composite had no effect on the results. All coefficients remain basically unchanged. Use of alternative measures of capital had a relatively negligible effect on the estimate of σ_0. However, the estimates of the individual effects of the various medical inputs did appear to be quite sensitive to alternative measures of capital. Clearly, further research is called for before the productivity of individual factors of production can be ascertained.

Attempts were made at various points in the investigation to add distribution parameters such as variables for low income and low education. It was found that in the cases considered, the explanatory power of the measures of the variables could not be improved upon by replacing them with the distribution parameters, and serious multicollinearity resulted when both forms were introduced simultaneously.

Discussion

Both models indicate that a 1 per cent increase in the quantity of medical services is associated with a reduction in mortality of about 0.1 per cent. Environmental conditions are a more important determinant of interstate variation in death rates. Among these, income and education play the greatest role. The effect of income on mortality is positive while that of education is negative. Urbanization is not important, but a number of labor force variables are. There is also some indication of harmful effects from cigarette smoking.

The positive coefficient of income is particularly interesting since it is contrary to gross relationships in most data. It should be borne in mind that the analysis holds constant the effects of medical care and education, variables that increase with income. Also, use of state averages, unlike use of individual observations or data grouped by income, greatly reduces the extent to which observed patterns are influenced by the tendency for some persons to have low income because their health is poor. Abstracting from these considerations, there are many reasons why income and mortality might be positively related.

We view persons as simultaneously determining consumption patterns, occupation, and life styles. As incomes rise, they might choose more adverse diets, faster cars, less exercise, et cetera. Also, occupations with less exercise, more strain, high risk of accident, et cetera might be selected in order to obtain higher income. The results of this study suggest that both occupation- and consumption-related factors may be important.

The education variable may also represent quite complex forces.

We do not know if we have isolated effects of the educational process or simply greater ability or willingness to learn. Even if what we have found does represent the effects of education, it is not clear whether general education or specific health training, such as in hygiene classes and exposure to school health programs, is relevant. There are many unanswered questions as to the patterns of care to which learning leads. The more educated may seek more preventive care, obtain medical care at earlier stages of an illness, have a better follow-up on drugs prescribed and referrals, or receive more continuous care. The last factor may be related to differences in the year-to-year variability of income between the more and less educated.

In comparisons among both developed and underdeveloped countries, Irma Adelman estimated the elasticity of the death rate with respect to the number of physicians per capita for specific age groups.[21] Her estimates of the impact of medical services on health are remarkably close to those in our study. Income, the rate of growth of income, and the proportion of the labor force employed outside agriculture were held constant. It seems likely that in international comparisons the number of physicians per capita is a good index of the total quantity of death-related medical services. Furthermore, since there is limited international factor mobility, it is probable that her estimates are relatively unbiased by her use of a single equation procedure. Her negative coefficient for income may reflect such factors as education, public health, and sanitation. Also, the effect of income may not be the same at all levels. She reports no significant difference between the coefficients for underdeveloped and developed countries, which may not hold true when education is added. Education has a positive sign in the Adelman study. Across countries, it may be associated with many of the factors with which income is associated across states. The income results with education included are not reported.

IMPLICATIONS AND CONCLUSIONS

One application of our results is to provide a possible explanation of recent trends in mortality in the United States. The age-adjusted death rate has not declined appreciably between about 1955 and 1965 (see Table 8-8), in spite of a substantial increase in the quantity of medical services produced per capita and probably some technological change as well. If we deflate national health expenditures by the Consumer

[21] See "An Econometric Analysis of Population Growth," *American Economic Review*, 53, June 1963, pp. 314–39.

TABLE 8-8

Contribution of Selected Medical Services and Environmental Factors to
Changes in the Age-adjusted Death Rate, 1955–65

	Percentage Change in Variable	Percentage Change in Mortality per Percentage Change in Variable	Percentage Change in Mortality
Actual change in U.S. death rate			−3.9%
National health expenditures per capita deflated by CPI for medical care	+35%	−0.1%	−3.5%
Median family income deflated by CPI for all items	+32%	+0.2%	+6.4%
Education	+17%	−0.2%	−3.4%
Cigarette consumption per capita	+18%	+0.1%	+1.8%

Source: U.S. Bureau of the Census, *Statistical Abstract of the United States, 1967,*
various tables.

Price Index for medical care, we find an increase in real expenditures
per capita of 35 per cent between 1955 and 1965. This alone would
lead us to expect a decline in the death rate of about 4 per cent. The
effect of the medical school variable over time cannot be similarly
derived, because its effects will be spread out and depend more on the
past rather than on the present growth of the schools. What, then,
has offset the expected decline? The answer is provided by the environmental factors, although a literal application of the estimated
coefficients to time series may not be fully justified. The growth of
education would have led to a decline of about 3 per cent. On the
other hand, changes in real family income would have increased mortality. With a literal application of the estimates, the effect of income is
6 per cent. However, occupation will tend to vary less with income
over time than in cross sections, because technological change also
contributes to changes in income. This suggests that a smaller estimate of the effects of income on changes in mortality is appropriate.
Changes in cigarette consumption per capita would have led to a
further increase of 2 per cent, although this is a case for which changes
over a longer period are clearly more appropriate. Our results, then,
would imply that adverse environmental factors have been offsetting
the advantages of increases in the quantity and quality of medical care.
We can estimate the effects of improvements in the effectiveness of
medical services as all changes not attributable to either changes in
the quantity of medical care or environment. Literal predictions based

on the variables in Table 8-8 would imply that in the period 1955–65 technological change reduced mortality by —3.9 minus 1.3 per cent, or a total of 5.2 per cent. Converted to an annual rate, this change is a change in mortality due to technology of 0.5 per cent per year. Allowing for the effects of medical schools and modifying the coefficient of income would produce an even smaller estimate of the contribution of technology change in the 1955–65 period. What may be an appropriate explanation since 1955 is not likely to be one for a longer period of time since in prior years the death rate fell precipitously. Unless the marginal effectiveness of medical care is substantially lower than in the past, one would have to infer that a slowdown in technological advance occurred.

It is also interesting to examine the implications of our results for white-nonwhite mortality differentials. In 1960, the white death rate was only 69 per cent of the nonwhite death rate when both are adjusted to the U.S. age distribution. Medical care spending and education would account for a large part of the difference, with small offsets from cigarette and possibly alcohol consumption. The application of the results on income to this problem seems highly questionable, since income may represent different variables at different ends of the income distribution. The color differential in mortality could be "explained" by our equations only if the predicted effect of income were omitted. We shall return to this point in a moment.

Some useful cost-benefit implications can be derived from the results. Dorothy P. Rice has estimated the economic cost of mortality using the present discounted value of future earnings as a measure of the loss of production to the economy. For 1963, she estimates these costs alternatively as $49.9 billion and $40.6 billion, depending on whether a 4 per cent or a 6 per cent rate of discount is used.[22] If the effect of a 1 per cent increase in medical expenditures is to reduce death rates by 0.1 per cent, as our estimate suggests, the benefit in increased production would be $40–50 million. Adding an equal percentage reduction in the loss from morbidity would bring the benefits to about $60–70 million. In 1963, however, national health expenditures were $32.9 billion, so that the costs of a 1 per cent increase in medical services would have been $329 million. While this comparison implies that costs exceed benefits, it should be noted that we have only considered economic losses due to the loss of productive time. No allowance has been made either for the loss of productivity due to

[22] Dorothy P. Rice, *Estimating the Cost of Illness*, U.S. Public Health Service Publication No. 947–6, May 1966, Tables 31 and 32.

illness or for the large psychic costs resulting from poor health. Also, the percentage effect of an across-the-board increase in the quantity of medical care may reduce morbidity losses by a very different percentage than mortality losses. We have examined the impact of variation in medical care generally. This type of cost-benefit comparison is relevant to a general increase in the quantity of medical care such as results from increased health insurance coverage. Specific programs may be able to select problems and areas with higher returns.

Statements regarding the merits of increments to educational spending relative to medical care can be made with less concern about the problems of benefit measurement. The effects of education on mortality are about double those of medical care, according to our estimates. Increases in education would presumably save medical resources as well. Yet a 1 per cent increase in the quantity of education involves only about one and one-half times the additional dollars. This would suggest that the tradeoff favors education, although again we need to know the relative effects on morbidity.[23,24] In view of the many other benefits of education, however, this result strongly suggests that the return on expenditures for additional education are far greater than on additional expenditures for medical care.

It is possible to integrate a great many of our findings, and in particular the observed effect of income on health, into a coherent, although somewhat conjectural, framework. Let us begin with the empirical observation that the gross relationship between health and income has the form H_T in Figure 8–1, ascending at a decreasing rate until it becomes approximately level over a wide range. This has been found to be the case for a large number of health measures, e.g., 365 minus the number of the disability days per person per year.[25] The beneficial

---

[23] The value of the effect on education of improvement in health attributable to an increase in medical care is likely to be much smaller than the saving in medical care due to an increase in education. See Irving Leveson, Doris Ullman, and Gregory Wassall, "Effects of Health on Education and Productivity," *Inquiry,* 6, December 1969, pp. 3–11.

[24] This comparison might overstate the merits of increasing education because forgone earnings of students may be greater than forgone earnings of medical patients. Also, to some extent, interstate differences in education may reflect interstate differences in native ability which would not be increased when education is increased over time.

[25] For example, see U.S. Public Health Service, *Medical Care, Health Status, and Family Income, United States,* National Center for Health Statistics Report, Series 10, No. 9, Washington, May 1964.

Our assumptions about the shape of H_T are derived from inspections of health measures individually. If each measure had a similar shape, but, as incomes

effects of medical care and education on health, both of which rise with income, are represented by H_{M+E}, which is monotonically increasing at perhaps a decreasing rate. H_T can be considered as resulting from H_{M+E} and the effects of factors other than medical care and education which are associated with income, H_Y. Alternatively, H_Y can be derived as a residual by subtracting H_{M+E} from H_T. In effect, we can consider H_Y to represent approximately the same factors as the income variable in our regressions. H_Y rises steadily and reaches a maximum at relatively low levels of income, declining continuously thereafter. The rising portion represents the effects of factors such as basic nutrition, sanitation, and housing, while the declining portion represents such factors as diet, exercise, and stress.[26]

This model is consistent with our finding of an adverse effect of income and also with the findings of Irma Adelman across countries, because of the unique income level of the United States. More generally, the model tends to explain the difference between our results and those of other studies concentrating on low income groups. It should also

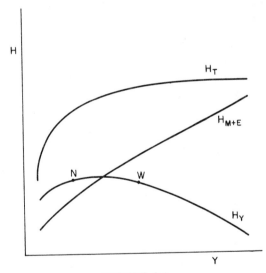

FIGURE 8-1
The Effects of Income, Education, and Medical Care on Health

rose, the weight in a combined health index shifted to measures that level off at higher incomes, the following remarks would hold only for mortality and not for health generally.

[26] If this is correct, then by fitting a monotonic relationship to H_Y one tends to underestimate the adverse effects of factors associated with income on health.

be noted that replacing the mean-income variable by the percentage of persons with low income would give a greater weight to the rising portion of the curve. When this was done, a smaller adverse effect of income was found.

Now consider the attempt to explain the white-nonwhite differential. We noted that a reconciliation could be made only if the predicted effects of income were not included. Suppose, however, that the average income of whites was at a point on H_Y such as W and those of nonwhites at N. Factors associated with income would then have both positive and negative effects on the differential. If these canceled, the reconciliation of the color difference would be succesful. If the income effect were not important in explaining the color differential, however, its impact on the total death rate ought to be much smaller than on white mortality. This view is supported by the results in Table 8-1.

At this point we are tempted to speculate that those factors which account for the declining portion of H_Y are also responsible for the higher death rates in the United States than in many European countries. Perhaps in that comparison, differences in the way people make a living, spend money, and allocate their time more than outweigh the effects of medical care and education. We might also expect that adverse effects of stress, exercise, and diet associated with income will not apply to infants. This model would therefore predict the negative association between income and infant mortality which has commonly been found. Again, the speculative nature of these remarks needs emphasis.

PART IV

SPATIAL VARIATIONS IN MORTALITY RATES

9

An Econometric Analysis of
Spatial Variations in Mortality Rates
by Race and Sex   *Morris Silver*

1. INTRODUCTION

The wish to measure the effects of income, schooling, and a variety of other variables upon mortality and to isolate their role in explaining the difference in mortality rates of whites and blacks in the United States is the primary factor motivating this study. To accomplish this we have applied multiple regression analysis to 1959–61 age-adjusted mortality rates by race and sex for states and standard metropolitan statistical areas (SMSA's). Questions about the effect of age adjustment on spatial patterns in mortality rates, about differences in the spatial patterns of age-specific mortality rates, and about the stability of mortality rates within and among geographic units over the 1959–61 period are dealt with in Appendix B.

Given the importance of and intrinsic interest in racial differences in mortality rates, it is surprising that attempts to subject them to econometric analysis have been so rare.[1] Brief summaries of the tech-

NOTE: I am indebted to Richard Auster, Michael Grossman, Gene Lewit, Jacob Mincer, Charlotte Muller, Kong-Kyun Ro, Mortimer Spiegelman, and especially to Victor Fuchs for many helpful comments.

[1] There have been many quantitative studies of mortality rates and other measures of health, but most of these are concerned only with the broad question of the influence of "social conditions" on health rather than with tests of specific economic or noneconomic hypotheses or estimation of specific parameters. A study by C. A. Moser and Wolf Scott (*British Towns,* London, 1961) is interesting and sophisticated, but its objectives—the quantification of social and economic differences among British towns—and variables are only slightly related to those of this study.

niques and findings of some of the few related prior studies in the field are presented below.

Adelman ran cross-country multiple regressions of thirty-four developed and underdeveloped countries, utilizing data falling in the period 1947–57.[2] The dependent variables are age-specific mortality rates and the independent variables include per capita income, the percentage rate of growth of per capita income, the percentage of the labor force employed outside agriculture, and the number of physicians per 10,000 inhabitants. Income elasticities are found to be negative in all cases and statistically significant up to age fifty, with values ranging from −0.14 for the forty–forty-four age group to −0.58 for the one–four age group. Higher percentages of the labor force outside agriculture tend to reduce mortality rates. Mortality rates are also found to be negatively correlated with the physician variable.

Fuchs chose states as his unit of observation and ran regressions for the years 1940, 1950, and 1960, utilizing both linear and logarithmic-linear unweighted and weighted forms (each state weighted by its population.)[3] In his first set of regressions the dependent variables are age-adjusted and infant mortality rates, while the independent variables include the number of physicians per capita, the rural percentage of the population, the nonwhite percentage of the population, the median income of families and unrelated individuals, the number of health personnel (including physicians) per capita, the foreign-born percentage of the population, and the median number of school years completed by the adult population. It is found that the percentage of nonwhites is positively correlated with age-adjusted mortality and is statistically significant. The coefficients of income for age-adjusted mortality are always *positive* and statistically significant in the 1960 regressions. On the other hand, they are predominantly *negative* for infant mortality, while also statistically significant. The other variables in the regressions do not exhibit consistent, statistically significant relationships with the dependent variables.

Auster, Leveson, and Sarachek utilized simultaneous equations techniques and the assumption of a Cobb-Douglas production function to estimate the effects of various medical services (e.g., physicians and drug expenditures per capita) on age-adjusted mortality rates across states for the entire population and for whites alone during 1959–61. Their study appears as chapter 8 of this volume.

[2] Irma Adelman, "An Econometric Analysis of Population Growth," *American Economic Review*, 53, June 1963, pp. 314–39.

[3] Victor R. Fuchs, "Some Economic Aspects of Mortality in the United States," New York, NBER, July 1965, pp. 13–27, mimeograph.

It is worth noting that both the Fuchs and the Auster, Leveson, and Sarachek study find strong positive relations across states between income and mortality, though not infant mortality, while Adelman observes the "traditional" inverse relationship across countries. A major objective of my study is to cast additional light on the relationship between income and mortality. In particular, an effort will be made to determine whether the relationship across SMSA's is different from that across states, how the income effect varies with sex and race, what the influence of the multicollinearity between income and schooling consists in, and whether the source of income (labor or nonlabor) is relevant.

In Section 2 the independent variables employed in the multiple regressions of Section 3 are classified and discussed. Race and sex differentials in mortality are examined in Section 4. The main findings are summarized and some concluding observations are offered in Section 5.

2. SOME VARIABLES DETERMINING MORTALITY BEHAVIOR

The factors believed to determine the mortality rate, which is taken as an inverse index of "health," and the corresponding statistical measures are classified as variables in the "consumer demand function for health" and "other" variables. The variables in the demand function are further classified as economic, informational, or taste. "Tastes" are interpreted to include health attitudes, perceptions, and motivations. Primary attention is directed to the roles of the economic and informational variables.

A complete list of all the variables examined in the course of this study is presented below. (Details on their construction and sources are given in Appendix A.) Variables marked by an asterisk were excluded from the final regressions featured in this article for various reasons explained in the text; exploratory regressions using them are available from the author on request.

Variables Explored in the Regression Analysis

A. Variables in the Explanatory Equations

Y(DDR)	Directly age-adjusted death rate (per 1,000 population) for all ages (1959–61, by color and sex)
Y'(IDR)	Indirectly age-adjusted death rate for all ages (1959–61, by race and sex)
X_1(MHWY)	Median income of husband-wife families standardized for the age of the head (1959, by color)

X'_1(MPY)	Median income of persons age fourteen and over with incomes (1959, by race and sex)
X''_1(MHWYD)	MHWY above its third quartile = 0; MHWY below its third quartile = actual MHWY (1959, by color)
X'''_1(%LT3T)	Per cent of husband-wife families with annual cash incomes less than $3,000, standardized for the age of the head (1959, by color)
X_{1L}(LABY)	Labor income of head of family or his wife (1959, by color)
X_{1NL}(NLABY)	Nonlabor income of head of family or his wife (1959, by color)
X_2(EARNR)	Weekly earnings rate of persons age fourteen and over in the experienced civilian labor force (1959, by color and sex)
X_3(MRTL)	Age-standardized per cent married with spouse present (1960, by race and sex)
X_4(FRTL)	Age-standardized (all ages) number of children ever born per 1,000 women ever married (1960, by color)
X_5(REGN)	South = 1; all other = 0
X_6(FB)	Ratio of foreign-born whites to native-born whites multiplied by 100 (1960, by sex)
X_7(MS)	Median number of years of school completed by persons age twenty and over (1960, by color and sex)
X_8(%RCC)	Per cent of persons in geographic unit residing in central cities (1960, by race)
X_9(%LAB)	Laborers except farm and mine workers as a per cent of all employed persons (1960, by race and sex)
X_{10}(%MWLFPC)	Per cent of married women with husband present and children under six who are in the labor force (1960, by color)
X_{11}(%MFG)	Per cent of employed persons in manufacturing (1960, by race and sex)
X_{12}(%BLK)	Per cent of population black (1960)
X_{13}(SEG)	Index of nonwhite residential segregation in SMSA's (1950)
X_{14}(ULCR)	Measure of psychological tensions: age-standardized death rate of persons age fourteen and over from ulcers of the stomach and duodenum (1959–61, color and sex, SMSA's only)
X'_{14}(ULCRD)	ULCR divided by age-standardized death rate from influenza and pneumonia (1959–61, by color and sex, SMSA's only)
X_{15}(ATMP)	Average annual temperature 1931–60 (SMSA's only)

X'_{15}(ATMP)^2	Square of annual average temperature 1931–60 (SMSA's only)
X_{16}(AHUM)	Average relative humidity in 1960 (SMSA's only)
X'_{16}(AHUM)^2	Square of average relative humidity in 1960 (SMSA's only)
X_{17}(DTMP)	Average daily maximum temperature minus average daily minimum temperature for 1960 (SMSA's only)
X_{18}(DHUM)	Absolute average daily deviation of relative humidity in 1960 (SMSA's only)
X_{19}(GASDR)	Density of automobile emissions (total consumption of gasoline divided by area of SMSA) expressed in rank form (1961–65, SMSA's only)
X'_{19}(GASDD)	GASDR above its median = 1; GASDR below its median = 0
X_{20}(ACSPR)	Arithmetic average concentration of suspended particulates expressed in rank form (1961–65, SMSA's only)
X'_{20}(ACSPD)	ACSPR above its median = 1; ACSPR below its median = 0
X_{21}(SO$_2$DR)	Density of sulfur dioxide emissions (total emissions of sulfur dioxide divided by area of SMSA) expressed in rank form (1961–65, SMSA's only)
X'_{21}(SO$_2$DR)	SO$_2$DR above its median = 1; SO$_2$DR below its median = 0
X_{22}(PHYS)	Employed physicians in medical practice per 10,000 population (1960)
X_{23}(%HOUS)	Per cent of housing units with 1.5 or more persons per room (1960, by color)
X_{24}(POPD)	Number of persons per square mile of land area in 1960
X_{25}(%FS)	Number residing outside the state and in the South in 1955 as a per cent of those five years old and over (1960, by color and sex, states only)
X_{26}(CIG)	Index of cigarette smoking in 1955 (by color and sex, states only)
X_{27}(WTRH)	Water hardness 1950–51 (states only)
X_{28}(HIGHW)	Per capita state and local expenditures on highways (1962)
X_{29}(WELF)	Per capita state and local expenditures on public welfare (1962)
X_{30}(HOSP)	Per capita state and local expenditures on hospitals (1962)
X_{31}(HLTH)	Per capita state and local expenditures on health services other than hospitals (1962)

X_{32}(POL)	Per capita state and local expenditures on police protection (1962)
X_{33}(FIRE)	Per capita state and local expenditures on fire protection (1962)
X_{34}(SAN)	Per capita state and local expenditures on sanitation including sewerage (1962)

B. Supplementary Variables

X'_8(%RUA)	Per cent of persons in state residing in urbanized areas (1960, by race and sex)
X_{24N}(TPOP)	Total population of geographic unit
X_{28}(UO)	Per cent of state's nonagricultural workers belonging to unions in 1953
X_{29}(RS)	State employment change from 1950 to 1960 due to its regional share

Variables in the Demand for Health

The application of demand (or choice) theory to health and the empirical estimation of income and relative cost elasticities is quite natural. Like the more conventional goods, health provides psychic income to the household and is, in part, acquired through the expenditure of scarce resources—money and time. Further, the "quantity" of health is to some degree subject to "rational" calculation, i.e., it is not rigidly determined by cultural, technical, biological, and genetic factors.[4]

ECONOMIC VARIABLES: COMMAND OVER GOODS AND SERVICES (INCOME).[5] Command over goods and services is represented mainly by a measure of family income (X_1). However, key results are checked by using a measure of individual income (X'_1). The emphasis placed on results for family income and the use of a somewhat unorthodox measure of family income (the age-standardized income of husband-wife families) are explained by a number of considerations. First, most individuals are members of families that pool their economic resources.

[4] See Michael Grossman, "The Demand for Health: A Theoretical and Empirical Investigation," NBER, forthcoming.

[5] Theoretically, it is possible that changes in the earnings rate (X_2) as distinct from changes in income may affect the demand for health. However, in the present sample income and earnings rate are highly correlated and exploratory regressions produced the symptoms of serious multicollinearity. Since income is, at least in principle, the more general measure of command over goods and services, and neither economic theory nor intuition leads to confident predictions about the sign of earnings rate coefficients, it was decided to exclude EARNR from the analysis.

Second, the expected long-run income of young single individuals is measured better by family income and, more specifically, by husband-wife income than by their actual current income. Third, the lifetime realized income of older persons whose marriage partner has died is measured better by husband-wife income than by their actual current individual (or family) income. Fourth, variables not included in the statistical model might increase the mortality rate in a geographic unit, with a consequent increase in the proportion of families in which the husband or wife is deceased. An increase in the proportion of such families would reduce average family income and cause its estimated coefficient to be biased. This, however, would not be the case for husband-wife income. Fifth, the use of an income measure that is based on age-standardized husband-wife income operates to adjust income for what might be termed nondiscretionary variations in family size. To explicitly adjust income for the number of children would introduce a bias if, as I believe, the number of children depends upon the income of the married couple.

It is usually assumed that the income elasticity of demand for health is positive (i.e., that health is a "superior good"), but this would not be the case if certain goods the consumption of which is adverse to health (e.g., automobile usage, cigarettes, and rich foods) have sufficiently high positive income elasticities. Of course, it is proper to speak of an income elasticity of demand for health only if the consumer is aware of the effects (positive or negative) of his consumption decisions upon his health—if the health consequences of consuming certain items are not widely understood or are regarded as unproven,[6] it is conceivable that the magnitude and even the sign of the estimated income elasticity might not accurately reflect the household's health intentions.

Yet another problem in the estimation of income elasticities of demand for health is the existence of a number of nonconsumption factors that are positively correlated with income and that might tend to reduce health status. Such factors include psychological tensions and pressures associated with earning higher incomes, certain ways in which higher incomes are earned (e.g., arduous, sedentary, or risky types of work), aspects of the occupational and industrial distribution, and, perhaps, a higher opportunity cost for time spent by the household in the production of health. This problem is dealt with in two ways: (1) the best available measures of the troublesome factors were included in the multiple regressions, and (2), in addition to regressions including

---

[6] A possible example is cigarette smoking before the Surgeon General's report.

total family income (X_1) and total individual income (X'_1), special regressions were run utilizing crude estimates of labor income (X_{1L}) and nonlabor income (X_{1NL}) as measures of command over goods and services, and elasticities obtained for each.

HEALTH INFORMATION. The inclusion of a measure of health information is needed to standardize the analysis of other variables and is of independent interest. The cost of realizing a given level of health declines as the amount of health information available to the household increases, hence the "law of demand" predicts a positive relationship between such information and health. The measure employed is schooling (X_7), which is perhaps the best available indicator of spatial differences in the extent and diffusion of information pertaining to health. In addition to being more likely to have received training in such special topics as personal hygiene, sanitation, and nutrition, persons with more schooling know better how to seek out and select appropriate health services. Schooling also reduces the costs of acquiring sources of psychic income other than health, and consequently it is not really clear what happens to the *relative cost* of health. Additional difficulties arise in interpreting the coefficient of schooling because schooling probably increases the taste for health and is itself less arduous and dangerous than market work.[7]

The inclusion of schooling in the regressions substantially increases the difficulty of interpreting the results for income. This is true for a variety of reasons: (1) schooling is an alternative measure of wealth; (2) income is one of the determinants of the level of schooling; (3) holding schooling constant, increases in income might in large part be due to people "working harder" or doing more dangerous work; (4) higher incomes may lead individuals to improve their health status by demanding additional health information (schooling). Thus it is important and useful to pay careful attention to income coefficients derived from estimating equations that exclude schooling.

TASTE VARIABLES:[8] MARITAL STATUS, FERTILITY, AND REGION.
Marital Status. It is widely believed that being unmarried in a society such as our own subjects the individual to psychological stresses that ultimately reduce his health status. However, differences in attitudes associated with marital status may actually affect choices between health and other goods. For example, it seems likely that a married person will

---

[7] I owe the latter point to Charlotte Muller.

[8] Inconclusive exploratory findings for two additional taste variables—migration from the South (X_{25}) and nativity (X_6)—led to their exclusion from the analysis.

place a higher relative value on his health than a single person because the former has loved ones to consider and, on the average, the welfare of loved ones is more strongly dependent on the married person's health than upon his other sources of satisfaction (including those that have an adverse effect upon health).[9]

While emphasis upon the above line of reasoning leads to the classification of marital status as a taste variable, it might also be classified as an economic variable because being married may lower the relative prices of a number of health-producing items (e.g., nursing services and proper nutrition), with the consequence that the demand for these items and ultimately for health is increased. X_3 is the measure of marital status employed.

Fertility. There are two reasons for including a measure of the fertility of women (X_4) in the analysis. First, since higher fertility rates increase maternal (and related) mortality rates, they may reflect a desire to substitute a larger number of children or more frequent coition for health. Second, the fertility rate might be an inverse index of "rational behavior"—that is, a high fertility rate might be indicative of the fact that an individual weights present satisfactions highly relative to future ones. Such a weighting system would tend to impair health and raise mortality rates (e.g., through a lesser inclination to take preventive measures or through longer delays in seeking medical care). However, in view of the possibility that higher incomes lead married couples to demand smaller families in order to improve their health status it is wise to examine income coefficients derived from estimating equations which exclude fertility.

Region. A regional dummy variable might reflect a variety of cultural factors affecting choices between health and other goods. The South–non-South dichotomy reflected in X_5 is probably the most relevant.

Other Variables[10]

RESIDENCE. Our cities are no longer the "graveyard of countrymen," but, as Peterson points out, while epidemics no longer decimate the

---

[9] On the other hand, Charlotte Muller reminds me that marriage may sometimes induce persons, in the interest of loved ones, to "work harder" and make other choices with adverse health effects.

[10] The following additional variables were excluded from the analysis because exploratory regressions failed to convincingly demonstrate their importance: per cent in manufacturing (X_{11}), per cent of laborers excluding farm and mine

cities, "air pollution, traffic, overcrowding, and the stress of urban life still present special hazards." [11] However, these negative factors may be partially or wholly offset by medical care that is of higher quality and is more readily available in emergency cases. While a priori considerations do not dictate the expected sign, it seems worthwhile to include the per cent residing in central cities (X_8) as an independent variable.

PER CENT OF BLACK POPULATION. The per cent of the geographic unit's population that is black (X_{16}) may be relevant for at least two reasons: (1) this percentage may be positively correlated with the extent of racial discrimination against blacks[12] and may also reflect preferential treatment of whites in the areas of education and public health services; and (2) it may be positively correlated with the mortality rate of whites (and of blacks) because it represents greater "exposure" to blacks who, for example, suffer higher rates of various communicable diseases.

PSYCHOLOGICAL PRESSURES. It is commonly believed that the types of activities and circumstances causing significant increases in average incomes give rise to or are accompanied by psychological tensions and pressures that, in a variety of ways, tend to reduce health and shorten life. The regression coefficient of a measure of these tensions would be of independent interest and the inclusion of such a variable would make the coefficient of income a purer measure of the consumption aspect of health.

Perhaps the best available index of such pressures are death rates from ulcers of the stomach and duodenum (X_{14}).[13] Unlike other diseases that are believed to be caused or aggravated by tension, ulcers are responsible for only a small fraction of all deaths. Unfortunately, spatial variations in the death rate from ulcers may reflect factors such as the quality and quantity of medical care and attitudes toward

---

workers (X_9), labor force participation of women with young children (X_{10}), residential segregation of blacks (X_{13}), overcrowded housing conditions (X_{23}), population density (X_{24}), and water hardness (X_{27}).

[11] William Peterson, *Population,* New York, 1961, p. 266.

[12] For references to the literature and some empirical evidence, see Gary S. Becker, *The Economics of Discrimination,* Chicago, 1957, pp. 98–99 and 104–107.

[13] See Gene Kaufman and Theodore D. Woolsey, "Sex Differences in the Trend of Mortality from Certain Chronic Diseases," *Public Health Reports,* 68, August 1953, pp. 761–68. The ulcer death rate was found to be positively correlated with family income for each of the four race-sex groups included in the study.

such care as well as differences in psychological tensions. A crude attempt is made to purge the ulcer death rate of its nontension dimensions by dividing X_{14} by the death rate from influenza and pneumonia. The resulting measure of tension is X'_{14}.

PHYSICIANS PER CAPITA. Employed physicians in medical practice per 10,000 population in 1960 (X_{22}) is taken to represent public health conditions and the availability of medical care in an area. However, in view of the fact that the level of income in an area plays an important role in determining both public health conditions and the availability of medical care, it is of the utmost importance to examine income coefficients derived from estimating equations that exclude physicians per capita.

CIGARETTE CONSUMPTION. There is some justification for classifying cigarette consumption as a variable in the demand for health because, as is well known, many individuals consciously substitute the pleasures of smoking for those flowing from better health. However, cigarette smoking has been classified as an "other" variable because its health consequences were not widely understood until recently. The measure employed is an index of cigarette smoking for 1955 (X_{26}).

CLIMATE. It has long been argued that climatic conditions have important effects on health.[14] Among the factors mentioned most frequently are average levels of temperature and relative humidity and their variability. Accordingly, measures of average temperature (X_{15}, X'_{15}), average relative humility (X_{16}, X'_{16}), the variability of temperature (X_{17}), and the variation of relative humidity (X_{18}) are included in the regressions.

AIR POLLUTION. Recently published data on various pollutants for sixty-five SMSA's with more than 40,000 manufacturing employees make possible an examination of the effects of air pollution in the context of a multivariate analysis for SMSA's. The published air pollution variables, in the form of ranks for 1961 (65 indicates the most severe pollution), refer to density of automobile emissions (X_{19}), concentration of suspended particulates (X_{20}, representing pollution from fuel burning, including motor vehicles, open burning, incinerators, manufacturing, etc.), and density of sulfur dioxide emissions (X_{21}). The ranked data are supplemented by the dummy pollution variables (X'_{19}–X'_{21}).

---

[14] For an elaborate discussion on this question and some empirical evidence, see Ellsworth Huntington, *Civilization and Climate,* New Haven, 1948, chapters 7–9.

3. REGRESSION ANALYSIS

Organization of the Regressions

The relationships discussed in Section 2 are investigated for each race-sex group by means of both ordinary least squares and two-stage least squares for states and SMSA's.[15] In the first stage, each of the independent variables considered "endogenous" is regressed upon the "exogenous" independent variables plus a number of "supplementary" variables intended to increase statistical efficiency. The second stage consists of replacing the actual values of the endogenous variables with their predicted values and estimating the desired parameters.

The use of two-stage least squares is justified by the possibility that it may mitigate problems like the following: (1) High mortality rates may lower family income and earnings if they are accompanied by or associated with high rates of work loss due to illness or injury and declines in productivity. (2) Payments made to persons *because* they are ill (e.g., certain veterans and public assistance payments) may dominate geographic variations in nonlabor income and at the same time reduce the variance in total income. (3) The coefficients of schooling and earnings would be biased if (a) high mortality rates, by reducing the period over which economic returns are expected to be earned, lowered the incentive to invest in formal education and in other activities that improve skills and move persons up the occupational ladder;[16] and (b) poor health reduced years of schooling by causing individuals to drop out of schools, or to be dropped, because of poor attendance or academic performance. (4) The coefficient of physicians per capita may be biased because "where health is poor, ceteris paribus, the demand for doctors [and other health-producing resources] will tend to be high."[17] (5) The coefficients of marital status and fertility may be biased because healthy persons are more likely to get married and have children than unhealthy ones. In addition, high fertility rates may be a deliberate response to high rates of child mortality which, in turn, are positively correlated with the mortality rate at all ages. (6) The coefficient of the ulcer death rate would be biased if a higher ulcer death rate merely reflected a generally unsatisfactory health situation.

[15] See J. Johnston, *Econometric Methods*, New York, 1963, chap. 9.

[16] The relationship between mortality rates and the incentive to invest in human capital is explored by Gary S. Becker in his *Human Capital: A Theoretical and Empirical Analysis, with Special Reference to Education*, New York, NBER, 1964, pp. 49–50.

[17] See essay by Auster, Leveson, and Sarachek in this volume.

In addition to mitigating simultaneous equation problems, the use of two-stage least squares may improve estimates of coefficients by compensating for measurement errors in a more weakly measured endogenous variable like family income, which is based upon recall during an interview and does not take account of differences in price levels among geographic units. However, because of numerous statistical difficulties, the two-stage least squares results are utilized as a check, while conclusions are based primarily on the results for ordinary least squares.

The dependent variables utilized in the regressions are 1959–61 directly age-adjusted mortality rates for all ages (DDR, Y).[18] It is well known that deficiencies in the census coverage of the black population introduce errors into their mortality rates.[19] However, the important question for the regression analysis that follows is whether the degree of underreporting varies systematically with our independent variables. According to Siegel,

> There is evidence from the reinterview studies of 1960 of poorer enumeration of housing units in very large cities and in rural areas than in small and moderate-size cities and in suburbs. No specific evidence from these studies is available by race relating city-size variations in coverage, whether of housing units or of persons in enumerated housing units; so we cannot say definitely whether the Negroes in the very large cities are more or less completely counted than Negroes in small or moderate-size cities or rural areas. There is a basis for suggesting that Negroes are counted most poorly in the very large cities in the fact that the 1960 enumeration in urban slums was more difficult and took longer than in other urban segments and in rural areas.[20]

To some extent, bias problems caused by underreporting may be mitigated by the inclusion in the regressions of the residence variable (X_8), the per cent of black population (X_{12}), and population density (X_{24}). Furthermore, a special regression for blacks including the absolute size of the black population as an independent variable did not perceptibly alter regression coefficients.

Since many of the variables included in the "black" regressions in actuality refer to nonwhites, these regressions are restricted to states and SMSA's in which at least 70 per cent of the nonwhites are blacks.

[18] Where possible, key results are checked by means of indirectly age-adjusted mortality rates for all ages (IDR, Y').

[19] See Appendix B.

[20] Jacob S. Siegel, "Completeness of Coverage of the Nonwhite Population in the 1960 Census and Current Estimates, and Some Implications," in *Social Statistics and the City,* Cambridge, Mass., 1968, p. 56.

The "full sample" regressions for SMSA's include fifty-nine SMSA's for blacks and ninety-nine for whites,[21] while the corresponding sample sizes for states are thirty-two and forty-eight. Differences in the specifications of state and SMSA regressions are due to the unavailability of certain independent variables for a given type of geographic unit and the statistical requirements of the two-stage least squares analysis.

The natural value weighted regressions (the weights being the square roots of the numbers of persons in a race-sex group) shown in Table 9-1 are the outcome of extensive experimentation. Key results have been checked by means of unweighted regressions and logarithmic regressions. In order to conserve space and avoid burdening the general reader with excessive detail, the exploratory regressions are omitted here and are available from the author upon request.

Results for Ordinary Least Squares

INCOME. Regression 1 provides little or no evidence of a negative relationship between family income (MHWY) and mortality. In the case of black males the income coefficients are negative but statistically insignificant, while the coefficients are *positive* and usually significant for the other race-sex groups. However, excellent reasons for stressing income coefficients derived from estimating equations that exclude schooling (MS), physicians per capita (PHYS), and fertility (FRTL) are provided by the a priori arguments of Section 2 and some relatively high observed intercorrelations between the variables. For example, (a) the simple correlation coefficients between MHWY and FRTL are —0.54 (whites) and —0.76 (blacks) for SMSA's, while the corresponding values for states are —0.80 and —0.94; (b) for SMSA's the simple correlation coefficients between MHWY and MS range from 0.25 (white females) to 0.85 (black males), with the corresponding range for states at 0.46 to 0.94; (c) the simple correlations between MHWY and PHYS are 0.49 (whites) and 0.46 (blacks) for SMSA's, while the corresponding state values are 0.73 and 0.83; (d) the correlations between FRTL and MS are negative and reach values of —0.74 (SMSA's) and —0.92 (states) for black females;[22] (e) the correlations between MS and PHYS range from 0.31 (white females) to 0.66

---

[21] In some SMSA's certain white independent variables actually refer to the total population, but this is only the case where nonwhites represent a trivial fraction of the total population.

[22] These correlations may reflect the fact that both schooling and fertility are indexes of the level of contraceptive knowledge.

(black males) for SMSA's, while the corresponding range for states is 0.27 to 0.80.[23]

When MS, PHYS, and FRTL are excluded (see regression 1*) the results tend to support the existence of a *negative* relationship.[24] While the state income coefficients for whites are positive (significant for white males), the remaining income coefficients are negative and approach or achieve statistical significance at conventional levels.[25] The income coefficients for black males are significantly lower (taking account of signs) than those for white males.[26] The observed differences in state and SMSA results for income, and certain other variables, probably cannot be attributed to differences in the regional coverage of the regressions.[27] However, while the exact cause of this difference remains unclear,[28] serious problems of interpretation are forestalled by the fact that, with the application of two-stage least squares analysis (white females) and the replacement of total income by labor and nonlabor income (white males), the income results for states and SMSA's bear

[23] Exploratory regressions for SMSA's reveal that the inclusion of PHYS raises the adjusted coefficient of determination for each of the race-sex groups while it substantially reduces the magnitudes of the MS regression coefficients and computed t values.

[24] There are reasons for believing that the effect of income varies with its level—for example, it may decline because technical considerations bring about a state of affairs in which the expenditure of an extra dollar will bring no increase in length of life. (In such a situation individuals might be expected to turn increasingly to "close" substitutes for length of life such as goods and services promoting physiological well-being within a fixed length of life.) In order to take account of this possibility experiments were carried out with a dummy income variable (X''_1) and the per cent of families below the "poverty line" of $3,000 ($X'''_1$). The results are tainted by multicollinearity problems and do not convincingly demonstrate the existence of differences in effect over the income ranges considered in the race-sex regressions.

[25] Comparisons reveal that when family income (MHWY) is replaced by individual income (MPY), the results often vary perceptibly but rarely dramatically.

[26] But see the white male results for nonlabor income. A complete set of significance tests is available from the author.

[27] The results of a state regression excluding states not represented in the SMSA regressions differ in detail but not in substance from those noted in the text.

[28] The simple correlations between MHWY and DDR, by race-sex groups, are shown below:

	WM	*WF*	*BM*	*BF*
State	.24	.50	−.39	−.59
SMSA	.07	.19	−.30	−.39

TABLE 9-1

Natural Value Weighted[a] Regressions of Age-adjusted Mortality Rates for All Ages on Various Independent Variables (SMSA's and States, 1959–61): Second Stage of Two-Stage Least Squares and Corresponding Results for Ordinary Least Squares Analysis

WHITE MALES

Independent Variable	Regression 1 — 99 Observations (2-SLS, SMSA)	Regression 1 — 99 Observations (OLS, SMSA)	Regression 1 — 48 Observations (2-SLS, State)	Regression 1 — 48 Observations (OLS, State)	Regression 1* — 99 Observations (2-SLS, SMSA)	Regression 1* — 99 Observations (OLS, SMSA)	Regression 1* — 48 Observations (2-SLS, State)	Regression 1* — 48 Observations (OLS, State)
MHWY X_1	0.0001 [0.059] (0.60)	0.0001 [0.059] (0.94)	0.0003 [0.201] (1.37)	0.0004 [0.268] (2.82)[d]	-0.0000 [-0.000] (-0.22)	-0.0002 [-0.119] (-2.54)[c]	0.0003 [0.201] (2.31)[c]	0.0002 [0.134] (2.43)[c]
NIABY X_{1NL}	—	—	—	—	—	—	—	—
LABY X_{1L}	—	—	—	—	—	—	—	—
MRTL X_3	-0.111 [-0.641] (-2.02)[c]	-0.091 [-0.527] (-5.22)[d]	0.026 [0.192] (0.38)	-0.028 [-0.209] (-0.80)	-0.054 [-0.313] (-1.68)	-0.093 [-0.538] (-5.46)[d]	0.042 [0.312] (0.92)	-0.034 [-0.254] (-1.08)
FRTL X_4	0.006 [1.066] (2.57)[c]	0.0009 [0.174] (2.95)[d]	-0.0006 [-0.164] (-0.58)	0.0002 [0.055] (0.69)	—	—	—	—
MS X_7	-0.095 [-0.091] (-0.48)	-0.204 [-0.196] (-3.05)[d]	-0.203 [-0.238] (-1.60)	-0.175 [-0.205] (-2.07)[c]	—	—	—	—

(continued)

TABLE 9-1 (continued)

		(1)	(2)	(3)	(4)	(5)	(6)	(7)	(8)
% RCC[b]	X_8	—	—	0.279 [0.009] (0.35)	-0.251 [-0.008] (-0.45)	—	—	-0.324 [-0.011] (-0.59)	-0.471 [-0.015] (-0.89)
% BLK[b]	X_{12}	0.093 [0.084] (4.08)[d]	0.047 [0.042] (6.56)[d]	0.009 [0.009] (0.98)	0.017 [0.018] (2.25)[e]	0.032 [0.029] (2.89)[d]	0.042 [0.038] (5.35)[d]	0.012 [0.013] (1.49)	0.018 [0.019] (2.36)[e]
ULCR	X_{14}	0.256 [0.248] (2.44)[e]	0.093 [0.090] (3.31)[d]	—	—	-0.016 [-0.015] (-0.18)	0.089 [0.086] (2.71)[d]	—	—
PHYS	X_{22}	0.041 [0.061] (1.13)	-0.015 [-0.021] (-1.42)	-0.052 [-0.074] (-0.68)	-0.014 [-0.020] (-0.43)	—	—	—	—
CIG[b]	X_{26}	—	—	0.012 [0.226] (2.25)[e]	0.011 [0.200] (2.57)[e]	—	—	0.014 [0.265] (3.21)[d]	0.011 [0.193] (2.67)[e]
Constant		2.46	16.03	7.31	8.21	15.31	17.90	2.29	8.66
R^2		0.280	0.584	0.445	0.511	0.139	0.396	0.397	0.433
$\bar{R}^2$		0.224	0.552	0.331	0.410	0.102	0.370	0.325	0.365

(continued)

TABLE 9-1 (continued)

WHITE MALES

Independent Variable	Regression 2 · 99 Observations (2-SLS, SMSA)	Regression 2 · 99 Observations (OLS, SMSA)	Regression 2 · 48 Observations (2-SLS, State)	Regression 2 · 48 Observations (OLS, State)	Regression 2* · 99 Observations (2-SLS, SMSA)	Regression 2* · 99 Observations (OLS, SMSA)	Regression 2* · 48 Observations (2-SLS, State)	Regression 2* · 48 Observations (OLS, State)
MHWY X_1	—	—	—	—	—	—	—	—
NLABY X_{1NL}	0.002 [0.336] (0.60)	-0.0002 [-0.034] (-0.75)	-0.002 [-0.298] (-1.53)	-0.0003 [-0.056] (-0.47)	-0.002 [-0.370] (-3.53)[d]	-0.0008 [-0.135] (-3.64)[d]	-0.002 [-0.280] (-2.14)[c]	-0.0007 [-0.131] (-1.72)
LABY X_{1L}	-0.0001 [-0.043] (-0.26)	0.0001 [0.043] (1.43)	0.0007 [0.338] (2.31)[d]	0.0005 [0.241] (3.07)[d]	0.0004 [0.170] (2.01)[c]	-0.0000 [-0.000] (-0.06)	0.0007 [0.338] (3.41)[d]	0.0004 [0.193] (2.79)[d]
MRTL X_3	-0.122 [-0.705] (-2.09)[c]	-0.099 [-0.570] (-5.33)[d]	-0.111 [-0.832] (-1.13)	-0.056 [-0.421] (-1.34)	-0.147 [-0.846] (-3.69)[d]	-0.119 [-0.684] (-6.34)[d]	-0.056 [-0.423] (-0.98)	-0.079 [-0.593] (-2.14)[c]
FRTL X_4	0.010 [1.976] (1.18)	0.0008 [0.155] (2.58)[d]	-0.0004 [-0.109] (-0.48)	0.0001 [0.027] (0.26)	—	—	—	—
MS X_7	0.075 [0.072] (0.21)	-0.206 [-0.199] (-3.10)[d]	0.005 [0.006] (0.03)	-0.147 [-0.172] (-1.67)	—	—	—	—

(continued)

TABLE 9-1 (continued)

		(1)	(2)	(3)	(4)	(5)	(6)	(7)	(8)
% RCC[b]	X_8	—	—	−0.480 [−0.016] (−0.54)	−0.489 [−0.016] (−0.59)	—	—	−0.981 [−0.032] (−1.69)	−0.792 [−0.026] (−1.50)
% BLK[b]	X_{12}	0.133 [0.121] (1.79)	0.046 [0.042][d] (6.48)	0.020 [0.021] (1.90)	0.020 [0.021][c] (2.51)	0.045 [0.041][d] (4.05)	0.043 [0.039][d] (5.60)	0.023 [0.024][c] (2.59)	0.022 [0.024][d] (2.92)
ULCR	X_{14}	0.259 [0.251][c] (2.45)	0.100 [0.097][d] (3.49)	—	—	0.170 [0.164] (1.74)	0.104 [0.101][d] (3.24)	—	—
PHYS	X_{22}	0.067 [0.099] (1.14)	−0.012 [−0.018] (−1.12)	−0.076 [−0.107] (−1.01)	−0.010 [−0.014] (−0.30)	—	—	—	—
CIG[b]	X_{26}	—	—	0.018 [0.333][d] (2.95)	0.012 [0.222][d] (2.80)	—	—	0.018 [0.334][d] (4.07)	0.013 [0.246][d] (3.34)
Constant		−12.82	16.82	15.14	10.69	21.12	19.50	9.28	11.80
R^2		0.282	0.591	0.492	0.528	0.245	0.444	0.478	0.489
$\bar{R}^2$		0.218	0.555	0.372	0.416	0.204	0.414	0.402	0.414

(continued)

TABLE 9-1 (continued)

WHITE FEMALES

Independent Variable	Regression 1 — 99 Observations (2-SLS, SMSA)	Regression 1 — 99 Observations (OLS, SMSA)	Regression 1 — 48 Observations (2-SLS, State)	Regression 1 — 48 Observations (OLS, State)	Regression 1* — 99 Observations (2-SLS, SMSA)	Regression 1* — 99 Observations (OLS, SMSA)	Regression 1* — 48 Observations (2-SLS, State)	Regression 1* — 48 Observations (OLS, State)
MHWY X_1	-0.002 [-1.782] (-0.77)	0.0003 [0.281] (3.48)[d]	-0.0000 [-0.000] (-0.03)	0.0003 [0.332] (4.54)[d]	-0.001 [-1.219] (-3.12)[d]	-0.0002 [-0.188] (-1.99)	-0.0001 [-0.111] (-0.93)	0.0001 [0.111] (0.73)
NLABY X_{1NL}	—	—	—	—	—	—	—	—
LABY X_{1L}	—	—	—	—	—	—	—	—
MRTL X_3	-0.116 [-0.978] (-1.50)	-0.097 [-0.820] (-7.47)[d]	-0.019 [-0.223] (-0.33)	-0.055 [-0.639] (-3.18)[d]	-0.147 [-1.238] (-5.25)[d]	-0.084 [-0.710] (-6.52)[d]	-0.088 [-1.025] (-4.51)[d]	-0.080 [0.938] (-5.05)[d]
FRTL X_4	-0.004 [-1.224] (-0.58)	0.0009 [0.275] (3.98)[d]	-0.0005 [-0.226] (-0.55)	0.0008 [0.361] (3.80)[d]	—	—	—	—
REGN[b] X_5	-2.635 [-0.061] (-0.95)	-0.349 [-0.008] (-2.86)[d]	-0.519 [-0.026] (-2.88)[d]	-0.346 [-0.017] (-3.36)[d]	-1.934 [-0.045] (-4.46)[d]	-0.666 [-0.015] (-3.75)[d]	-0.436 [-0.022] (-2.64)[c]	-0.334 [-0.004] (-2.24)[c]
MS X_7	-0.037 [-0.056] (-0.09)	-0.262 [-0.402] (-5.07)[d]	-0.356 [-0.721] (-2.32)[c]	-0.251 [-0.508] (-4.95)[d]	—	—	—	—

(continued)

TABLE 9-1 (continued)

		(1)	(2)	(3)	(4)	(5)	(6)	(7)	(8)
% RCC[b]	X₈	—	—	0.161 [0.009] (0.30)	−0.278 [−0.016] (−0.95)	—	—	−0.232 [−0.013] (−0.55)	−0.205 [−0.011] (−0.52)
% BLK[b]	X₁₂	0.068 [0.097] (1.56)	0.023 [0.033] (3.71)[d]	0.009 [0.015] (1.19)	0.012 [0.021] (2.44)[c]	0.080 [0.115] (3.63)[d]	0.031 [0.044] (3.47)[d]	0.014 [0.024] (1.88)	0.011 [0.019] (1.58)
ULCR	X₁₄	−0.381 [−0.172] (−0.35)	0.103 [0.047] (2.19)[c]	—	—	−0.007 [−0.003] (−0.02)	0.148 [0.067] (2.16)[c]	—	—
PHYS	X₂₂	−0.046 [−0.109] (−0.83)	−0.027 [−0.063] (−3.15)[d]	−0.018 [−0.041] (−0.28)	0.001 [0.002] (0.05)	—	—	—	—
CIG[b]	X₂₆	—	—	0.014 [0.111] (1.88)	0.012 [0.097] (2.22)[c]	—	—	0.007 [0.053] (0.83)	−0.0004 [−0.003] (−0.05)
WELF[b]	X₂₉	—	—	−0.005 [−0.023] (−1.00)	−0.010 [−0.050] (−3.19)[d]	—	—	−0.005 [−0.023] (0.99)	−0.010 [−0.049] (−2.24)[c]
Constant		38.89	12.56	11.65	7.79	24.59	13.06	11.56	10.62
R^2		0.472	0.798	0.746	0.860	0.457	0.526	0.647	0.675
$\bar{R}^2$		0.425	0.780	0.677	0.823	0.428	0.501	0.585	0.618

(continued)

TABLE 9-1 (continued)

WHITE FEMALES

Independent Variable	Regression 2 — 99 Observations (2-SLS, SMSA) (OLS, SMSA)	Regression 2 — 48 Observations (2-SLS, State) (OLS, State)	Regression 2* — 99 Observations (2-SLS, SMSA) (OLS, SMSA)	Regression 2* — 48 Observations (2-SLS, State) (OLS, State)
MHWY X_1	—	—	—	—
NLABY X_{1NL}	-0.0006 [-0.479] (-0.55); 0.0004 [0.319] (6.26)[d]	0.0001 [0.094] (0.20); 0.0004 [0.377] (4.82)[d]	-0.003 [-1.996] (-2.44)[c]; 0.0002 [0.160] (1.81)	-0.0000 [-0.000] (-0.09); 0.0002 [0.188] (1.84)
LABY X_{1L}	0.012 [1.617] (0.99); -0.0001 [0.014] (-0.38)	-0.0003 [-0.049] (-0.57); -0.0000 [-0.000] (-0.11)	0.0000 [0.000] (0.03); -0.001 [-0.195] (-5.17)[d]	-0.0005 [-0.082] (-1.29); -0.0005 [-0.082] (-1.69)
MRTL X_3	-0.454 [-3.836] (-1.11); -0.096 [-0.813] (-7.16)[d]	0.016 [-0.190] (-0.28); -0.053 [-0.613] (-3.10)[d]	-0.190 [-1.602] (-4.41)[d]; -0.083 [-0.704] (-7.17)[d]	-0.088 [-1.031] (-4.55)[d]; -0.081 [-0.942] (-5.24)[c]
FRTL X_4	0.022 [6.699] (1.06); 0.0007 [0.214] (3.03)[d]	-0.0004 [-0.180] (-0.42); 0.0007 [0.316] (3.53)[d]	—	—
REGN[b] X_5	—	-0.522 [-0.026] (-2.88)[d]; -0.342 [-0.017] (-3.44)[d]	-2.987 [-0.069] (-3.29)[d]; -0.455 [-0.011] (-2.74)[d]	-0.443 [-0.022] (-2.67)[c]; -0.329 [-0.016] (-2.28)[c]
MS X_7	-0.213 [-0.327] (-0.86); -0.276 [-0.423] (-5.25)[d]	-0.360 [-0.729] (-2.33)[c]; -0.249 [-0.505] (-5.01)[d]	—	—

(continued)

TABLE 9-1 (continued)

		(1)	(2)	(3)	(4)	(5)	(6)	(7)	(8)
% RCC[b]	X₈	—	—	0.033 [0.002] (0.06)	-0.366 [-0.021] (-1.25)	—	—	-0.299 [-0.017] (-0.70)	-0.334 [-0.019] (-0.80)
% BLK[b]	X₁₂	0.207 [0.296] (1.12)	0.011 [0.016] (2.25)[c]	0.012 [0.020] (1.36)	0.014 [0.025] (2.85)[d]	0.117 [0.168] (3.27)[d]	0.025 [0.355] (3.08)[d]	0.017 [0.030] (2.17)[c]	0.015 [0.027] (2.17)[c]
ULCR	X₁₄	2.008 [0.909] (1.29)	0.109 [0.049] (2.28)[c]	—	—	-0.082 [-0.037] (-0.27)	0.135 [0.061] (2.18)[c]	—	—
PHYS	X₂₂	0.096 [0.226] (0.85)	-0.024 [-0.056] (-2.74)[d]	-0.006 [-0.014] (-0.09)	0.005 [0.012] (0.25)	—	—	—	—
CIG[b]	X₂₆	—	—	0.015 [0.118] (1.96)	0.013 [0.100] (2.33)[c]	—	—	0.008 [0.065] (1.01)	0.001 [0.009] (0.16)
WELF[b]	X₂₉	—	—	-0.005 [-0.025] (-1.07)	-0.009 [-0.047] (-2.99)[d]	—	—	-0.005 [-0.024] (-1.01)	-0.009 [-0.043] (-2.99)[d]
Constant		-30.05	12.19	11.03	7.74	33.26	12.04	11.49	10.44
R^2		0.472	0.788	0.749	0.869	0.467	0.619	0.656	0.703
$\bar{R}^2$		0.425	0.770	0.672	0.829	0.432	0.594	0.588	0.642

(continued)

TABLE 9-1 (continued)

BLACK MALES

Independent Variable	Regression 1				Regression 1*			
	59 Observations (2-SLS, SMSA) (OLS, SMSA)		32 Observations (2-SLS, State) (OLS, State)		59 Observations (2-SLS, SMSA) (OLS, SMSA)		32 Observations (2-SLS, State) (OLS, State)	
MHWY X_1	−0.0005 [−0.153] (−0.55)	−0.0001 [−0.031] (−0.16)	−0.0002 [−0.058] (−0.23)	−0.0000 [−0.000] (−0.03)	−0.001 [−0.307] (−3.50)[d]	−0.0009 [−0.276] (−4.49)[d]	−0.001 [−0.347] (−2.45)[c]	−0.001 [−0.318] (−2.92)[d]
NLABY X_{1NL}	—	—	—	—	—	—	—	—
LABY X_{1L}	—	—	—	—	—	—	—	—
MRTL X_3	−0.070 [−0.262] (−0.32)	−0.154 [−0.580] (−3.22)[d]	−0.189 [−0.857] (−1.22)	−0.281 [−1.277] (−3.71)[d]	0.065 [0.247] (0.45)	−0.181 [−0.683] (−3.72)[d]	−0.243 [−1.104] (−1.76)	−0.289 [−1.312] (−3.98)[d]

(continued)

TABLE 9-1 (continued)

		(1)	(2)	(3)	(4)	(5)	(6)	(7)	(8)
MS	X_7	−0.470 [−0.280] (−0.66)	−0.550 [−0.328] (−1.81)	−0.894 [−0.541] (−2.05)[c]	−0.841 [−0.509] (−2.86)[d]	—	—	—	—
% RCC[b]	X_8	—	—	1.911 [0.078] (1.06)	1.567 [0.064] (1.15)	—	—	1.629 [0.066] (0.87)	0.729 [0.029] (0.49)
ULCR	X_{14}	0.408 [0.285] (2.95)[d]	0.135 [0.095] (2.99)[d]	—	—	0.369 [0.258] (2.74)[c]	0.130 [0.091] (2.61)[c]	—	—
PHYS	X_{22}	−0.074 [−0.087] (−0.62)	−0.056 [−0.067] (−1.49)	0.065 [0.061] (0.47)	−0.059 [−0.056] (−0.65)	—	—	—	—
Constant		21.27	27.15	27.91	33.65	11.60	26.71	28.91	31.38
R^2		0.246	0.505	0.380	0.607	0.218	0.376	0.280	0.461
$\bar{R}^2$		0.175	0.458	0.261	0.531	0.175	0.342	0.203	0.404

(continued)

TABLE 9-1 (continued)

BLACK MALES

Independent Variable	Regression 2				Regression 2*			
	59 Observations		32 Observations		59 Observations		32 Observations	
	(2-SLS, SMSA)	(OLS, SMSA)	(2-SLS, State)	(OLS, State)	(2-SLS, SMSA)	(OLS, SMSA)	(2-SLS, State)	(OLS, State)
MHWY X_1	—	—	—	—	—	—	—	—
NLABY X_{1NL}	-0.004 [-0.333] (-0.45)	0.002 [0.180] (2.40)[c]	0.002 [0.140] (0.50)	-0.003 [-0.306] (-1.92)	-0.0005 [-0.045] (-0.62)	-0.0006 [-0.056] (-0.31)	-0.0004 [-0.037] (-0.30)	
LABY X_{1L}	-0.0002 [-0.043] (-0.20)	-0.0006 [-0.130] (-1.52)	-0.0004 [-0.078] (-0.48)	-0.0007 [-0.152] (-1.76)	-0.001 [-0.022] (-3.56)[d]	-0.001 [-0.275] (-2.01)	-0.001 [-0.255] (-2.39)[c]	
MRTL X_3	-0.021 [-0.078] (-0.08)	-0.107 [-0.405] (-2.24)[c]	-0.169 [-0.768] (-1.06)	-0.254 [-1.153] (-3.35)[d]	-0.169 [-0.639] (-3.20)[d]	-0.076 [-0.286] (-0.43)	-0.217 [-0.986] (-1.35)	-0.272 [-1.232] (-3.31)[d]

(continued)

TABLE 9-1(continued)

MS X_7	−0.351 [−0.209] (−0.45)	−0.422 [−0.251] (−1.45)	−0.912 [−0.552][c] (−2.06)[c]	−0.876 [−0.530] (−3.05)[d]	—	—	—	—
% RCC[b] X_8	—	—	2.486 [0.101] (1.20)	2.426 [0.099] (1.69)	—	—	1.842 [0.075] (0.92)	0.961 [0.392] (0.60)
ULCR X_{14}	0.461 [0.322][c] (2.40)[c]	0.117 [0.082] (2.72)[d]	—	—	0.450 [0.315] (3.08)[d]	0.125 [0.087] (2.46)[c]	—	—
PHYS X_{22}	0.078 [0.092] (0.20)	−0.116 [−0.138] (−2.77)[d]	−0.014 [−0.014] (−0.07)	−0.129 [−0.123] (−1.31)	—	—	—	—
Constant	17.90	23.84	26.32	31.38	20.36	25.94	27.04	29.99
R^2	0.248	0.566	0.389	0.642	0.244	0.380	0.283	0.466
$\bar{R}^2$	0.161	0.516	0.242	0.556	0.188	0.334	0.177	0.387

(continued)

TABLE 9-1 (continued)

BLACK FEMALES

Independent Variable	Regression 1 — 59 Observations (2-SLS, SMSA) (OLS, SMSA)	Regression 1 — 32 Observations (2-SLS, State) (OLS, State)	Regression 1* — 59 Observations (2-SLS, SMSA) (OLS, SMSA)	Regression 1* — 32 Observations (2-SLS, State) (OLS, State)
MHWY X_1	0.0008 [0.330] (1.49) 0.0005 [0.206] (2.29)ᵉ	0.001 [0.470] (1.36) 0.0007 [0.274] (2.79)ᵈ	−0.0007 [−0.289] (−3.23)ᵈ −0.0006 [−0.248] (−3.90)ᵈ	−0.0006 [−0.235] (−1.57) −0.0004 [−0.159] (−1.28)
NLABY X_{1NL}	— —	— —	— —	— —
LABY X_{1L}	— —	— —	— —	— —
MRTL X_3	0.125 [0.556] (0.53) −0.078 [−0.344] (−2.87)ᵈ	−0.151 [−0.815] (−1.82) −0.140 [−0.757] (−4.24)ᵈ	−0.031 [−0.136] (−0.82) −0.075 [−0.331] (−2.89)ᵈ	−0.085 [−0.459] (−1.76) −0.113 [−0.609] (−3.21)ᵈ
FRTL X_4	−0.004 [−0.830] (−1.13) −0.0001 [−0.023] (−0.16)	0.0008 [0.267] (0.45) 0.0002 [0.067] (0.35)	—	—

(continued)

TABLE 9-1 (continued)

REGN[b]	X_5	—	—	0.899 [0.060] (0.85)	0.457 [0.031] (1.25)	—	—	−0.034 [−0.002] (−0.05)	0.256 [0.017] (0.49)
MS	X_7	−2.465 [−2.142] (−1.65)	−0.861 [−0.748] (−3.87)[d]	−0.744 [−0.687] (−1.80)	−0.728 [−0.672] (−4.00)[d]	—	—	—	—
% RCC[b]	X_3	—	—	1.908 [0.109] (1.36)	1.447 [0.083] (1.98)	—	—	1.082 [0.062] (0.94)	0.523 [0.030] (0.55)
ULCR	X_{14}	0.093 [0.028] (0.40)	0.081 [0.024] (1.28)	—	—	0.374 [0.111] (1.71)	0.140 [0.042] (1.61)	—	—
PHYS	X_{22}	0.044 [0.071] (0.20)	−0.075 [−0.121] (−3.17)[d]	−0.194 [−0.249] (−1.83)	−0.144 [−0.185] (−3.01)[d]	—	—	—	—
WELF[b]	X_{29}	—	—	−0.032 [−0.094] (−3.25)[d]	−0.036 [−0.104] (−5.31)[d]	—	—	−0.032 [−0.092] (−2.68)[e]	−0.031 [−0.090] (−2.94)[d]
Constant		31.69	21.44	17.30	20.40	13.81	16.26	15.39	16.00
R^2		0.350	0.676	0.723	0.870	0.160	0.293	0.472	0.570
$\bar{R}^2$		0.275	0.639	0.626	0.825	0.114	0.254	0.370	0.487

(continued)

TABLE 9-1 (continued)

BLACK FEMALES

Independent Variable	Regression 2				Regression 2*			
	59 Observations		32 Observations		59 Observations		32 Observations	
	(2-SLS, SMSA)	(OLS, SMSA)	(2-SLS, State)	(OLS, State)	(2-SLS, SMSA)	(OLS, SMSA)	(2-SLS, State)	(OLS, State)
MHWY X_1	—	—	—	—	—	—	—	—
NLABY X_{1NL}	0.007 [2.219] (1.33)	0.0008 [0.269] (2.99)[d]	0.001 [0.354] (1.26)	0.0008 [0.258] (2.89)[d]	0.002 [0.773] (2.82)[d]	0.0003 [0.101] (1.04)	0.0002 [0.064] (0.32)	0.0002 [0.064] (0.70)
LABY X_{1L}	−0.039 [−2.960] (−1.15)	−0.0006 [−0.046] (−0.96)	0.002 [0.161] (0.88)	0.0000 [0.000] (0.05)	0.010 [−0.742] (−4.00)[d]	−0.003 [−0.214] (−4.41)[d]	−0.003 [−0.218] (−2.24)[c]	−0.003 [−0.176] (−2.82)[d]
MRTL X_3	−0.075 [−0.331] (−1.00)	−0.095 [−0.422] (−3.39)[d]	−0.153 [−0.827] (−1.81)	−0.147 [−0.793] (−4.30)[d]	−0.386 [−1.717] (−3.83)[d]	−0.133 [−0.589] (−4.65)[d]	−0.176 [−0.952] (−2.63)[c]	−0.168 [−0.908] (−4.34)[d]
FRTL X_4	−0.006 [−1.267] (−1.55)	−0.0001 [−0.023] (−0.22)	0.0008 [0.267] (0.45)	0.0002 [−0.067] (0.43)	—	—	—	—
REGN[b] X_5	—	—	1.239 [0.083] (0.95)	0.324 [0.022] (0.81)	—	—	−0.356 [−0.024] (−0.56)	−0.067 [−0.005] (−0.14)

(continued)

TABLE 9-1 (concluded)

MS	X_7	1.362 [1.183] (0.38)	−0.874 [−0.760] (−4.01)ᵈ	−0.719 [−0.664] (−1.70)	−0.711 [−0.656] (−3.86)ᵈ	—	—	—
% RCCᵇ	X_8	—	—	2.293 [0.131] (1.38)	1.264 [0.072] (1.65)	—	−0.008 [−0.005] (−0.01)	−0.264 [−0.015] (−0.29)
ULCR	X_{14}	4.387 [1.306] (1.19)	0.110 [0.033] (1.72)	—	—	1.334 [0.397] (4.12)ᵈ	0.196 [0.058] (2.44)ᶜ	—
PHYS	X_{22}	0.500 [0.799] (1.12)	−0.055 [−0.089] (−2.18)ᶜ	−0.263 [−0.339] (−1.40)	−0.121 [−0.156] (−2.20)ᶜ	—	—	—
WELFᵇ	X_{29}	—	—	−0.031 [−0.090] (−2.96)ᵈ	−0.036 [−0.104] (−5.29)ᵈ	—	−0.032 [−0.094] (−2.86)ᵈ	−0.030 [−0.086] (−3.08)ᵈ
Constant		41.34	21.69	16.97	20.52	24.29	19.91	18.85
R^2		0.367	0.697	0.725	0.874	0.332	0.537	0.657
$\bar{R}^2$		0.280	0.655	0.613	0.823	0.283	0.426	0.575

Note: Two sets of regressions are shown, with the second identified by an asterisk to indicate omission of MS, PHYS, and FRTL. 2-SLS indicates results from the second stage of a two-stage least squares analysis. OLS indicates results from an ordinary least squares analysis. The regression coefficient appears first, followed by the elasticity at means, in brackets, and the computed *t* values, in parentheses.

ᵃ The weights are the square roots of the populations of the race-sex groups.

ᵇ Exogenous variable.

ᶜ The coefficient is statistically significant at the .05 level of significance.

ᵈ The coefficient is statistically significant at the .01 level of significance.

a closer resemblance.[29] The MHWY elasticities of the mortality rate derived from regression 1* range from −0.12 (white males) to −0.28 (black males) for SMSA's, while the range for states is 0.13 (white males) to −0.32 (black males).

The fact that health-producing goods and services consumed by less affluent households are sometimes paid for directly (by charity) or indirectly (by taxes) by more affluent households might produce a positive correlation between income and the "cost" of health. Such a correlation would cause underestimation of income regression coefficients that might be especially severe for blacks. In order to quantify this type of bias, I ran experimental black regressions that included white family income as well as other regressions that included a variety of public expenditure variables. The coefficients of white income have the expected negative signs (not significant), but the inclusion of white family income does not materially alter the coefficients of black income. The coefficients of the public expenditure variables are usually negative, but their inclusion has little or no systematic impact upon the black MHWY coefficients.

Bias in the estimated coefficients, especially the income coefficient, may have resulted from the failure to adjust the income figures for price level differences among geographic units at a given time. Unfortunately, the 1959 crude price data are available for only fifteen of the SMSA's included in the white and black regressions.[30] The reader may wish to use the results of regressions (excluding MS, PHYS, and FRTL) for these fifteen SMSA's to roughly gauge the magnitude of bias in the full sample income coefficients. In the case of white males the coefficient of "money" MHWY is −0.0003, while that of "real" MHWY is −0.0005; for white females the comparable figures are −0.0005 and −0.0007, for black males, −0.0017 and −0.0023, and for black females, −0.0009 and −0.0015.

Certain nonconsumption factors cause the "pure" income effect to be underestimated by simultaneously being correlated positively with income and tending to reduce health status, as pointed out in Section 2. To some extent the analysis has already been standardized for such factors by including ULCR, %MFG, %LAB, EARNR, %RCC, and

[29] It should be noted that the state income results already resemble those for SMSA's in that the exclusion of MS, PHYS, and FRTL reduces the algebraic values of the regression coefficients.

[30] The source of the price data is Helen H. Lamale and Margaret S. Stotz, "The Interim City Worker's Family Budget," *Monthly Labor Review*, August 1960, Table 2.

POPD in the regressions. However, at this point an attempt is made to obtain direct evidence on this question by replacing total family income (MHWY) by crude estimates of its labor (LABY) and nonlabor (NLABY) components. In regressions 2 and 2* for white males the coefficients of NLABY are negative in every case (approaching or achieving significance when MS, FRTL, and PHYS are excluded), while the coefficients of LABY are either positive (significant for states) or negative, but smaller in magnitude than the coefficient of NLABY.

These results are consistent with the view that for white males the observed coefficients of total family income represent a compromise between the favorable health effects of a "pure" increase in income and the unfavorable (or less favorable) health effects of increases in earnings resulting from "working harder" and doing more dangerous or sedentary types of work. On the other hand, for reasons that are uncertain, the results for the other race-sex groups tend to be unstable and the differences in labor and nonlabor coefficients do not lend themselves to meaningful interpretations.[31] It is important to note that when the comparison is between the white male coefficient for NLABY and the black male coefficient for MHWY, the observed racial income differential is considerably narrowed.

SCHOOLING (MS). There are difficulties in disentangling the health effects of schooling and income, but the regression coefficients of schooling consistently have the expected negative sign and often achieve statistical significance. The schooling elasticities derived from regression 1 are among the largest for each race-sex group, ranging from −0.20 (white males) to −0.75 (black females) for SMSA's.

Exploratory regressions reveal that even after account has been taken of MHWY, FRTL (a measure of contraceptive knowledge), and PHYS (reflecting the availability of medical care), the inclusion of MS increases (sometimes materially) the adjusted coefficients of determination. Tentatively, it may be concluded that health information plays an important role in determining mortality. Further, while increases in the demand for medical services and in the level of contraceptive knowledge may be important channels through which schooling exerts its influence, they are not the only channels.

MARITAL STATUS (MRTL). The regression coefficients of MRTL

[31] In this connection it must be noted that not only is our NLABY variable a crude estimate of "nonlabor income" but nonlabor income is itself a crude estimate of "pure" income. Capital gains, for example, may be achieved by means of difficult and anxiety-provoking work.

have the expected negative sign and typically are statistically significant. The marital status elasticities derived from regression 1 are among the largest for each race-sex group, ranging from —0.34 (black females) to —0.82 (white females).

FERTILITY (FRTL). The coefficients of FRTL have the expected positive sign, but consistent statistical significance is achieved only for white females.[32] The elasticities for white females are relatively high: 0.28 (SMSA's) and 0.36 (states). The failure of FRTL for black females is probably explained by its high correlation with schooling (—0.74 for SMSA's)[33]—exploratory regressions reveal that when MS is excluded the coefficient for black females is positive and significant.

The relative weakness of the FRTL results for males[34] casts doubt on the view that fertility can be regarded as an inverse index of "rational behavior" (see Section 2).

REGION (REGN). The coefficients for white females are negative and significant while those for black females are positive and sometimes significant in exploratory regressions for SMSA's.[35] The results suggest that residence in the South reduces the mortality rate of white women while it increases the rate for black women.

RESIDENCE (%RCC). The results for %RCC weakly suggest that for blacks the negative health aspects of residence in the central cities of SMSA's outweigh the positive aspects.[36]

PER CENT OF BLACK POPULATION (%BLK). The coefficients of %BLK are positive and significant for whites, but this variable is ex-

---

[32] The finding for white females is consistent with a recent study making use of data on deaths and various socioeconomic characteristics of individuals. The study found a positive association between mortality ratios, standardized for age and education, and fertility for white females. See Evelyn M. Kitagawa, "Social and Economic Differentials in Mortality in the United States, 1960," paper prepared for a session on socioeconomic differentials in mortality of the General Assembly and Conference of International Union for Scientific Study of Population, London, September 3–11, 1969.

[33] The corresponding correlation for white females is only — 0.17. The basis for the racial difference in the correlation between fertility and schooling is uncertain, but a racial difference in the correlation between the levels of schooling and contraceptive knowledge and practice is suspected.

[34] FRTL is excluded from the estimating equation for black males because exploratory regressions show that its coefficient is negative and very insignificant even when MS is excluded.

[35] The REGN variable is excluded from the male regressions because exploratory regressions reveal that the coefficients for white males fluctuate in sign and are insignificant, while those for black males are positive but never significant.

[36] The results for whites are mixed. While the state coefficients are *negative,* those observed in exploratory regressions for SMSA's are *positive.*

cluded from the black regressions because exploratory regressions reveal that its coefficients, while positive, are extremely insignificant. The basis for the racial difference in the impact of %BLK is uncertain, but it should be noted that in the case of blacks %BLK is highly correlated across SMSA's with MHWY (-0.67) and MS (-0.70).[37]

PSYCHOLOGICAL TENSION (ULCR). The coefficients of ULCR take the expected positive sign and are highly significant for males.[38] The estimated ULCR elasticities derived from regression 1 are relatively high: 0.09 (for both white and black males).

PHYSICIANS PER CAPITA (PHYS). The coefficients of PHYS have the expected negative sign, except for state data on white females.[39] That statistical significance is achieved only for females may indicate that geographic variations in the availability of medical care during childbirth significantly affect female health.

CIGARETTE SMOKING (CIG). The results for the cigarette variable provide additional evidence of a positive relationship between smoking and mortality. The elasticity of 0.20 for white males is among the highest in the study.[40]

PUBLIC WELFARE (WELF). The coefficients of WELF have the ex-

---

[37] The corresponding correlation coefficients for whites are 0.14 for MHWY and -0.01 (males) and -0.04 (females) for MS.

[38] ULCR rather than ULCRD (the ratio of the ulcer death rate to the death rate from influenza and pneumonia) is chosen to measure psychological tensions because exploratory regressions for SMSA's reveal that (1) the coefficient of ULCR always has the expected positive sign while the coefficient of the "deflated" ulcer variable is negative for black males, (2) computed t values are larger for the undeflated ulcer variable, and (3) the coefficients of multiple determination are somewhat larger when ULCR is utilized. Further, a tension variable is needed mainly to standardize the results for income, and in this respect the undeflated variable seems to have the advantage—the income coefficients are consistently negative and, with the exception of black females, the negative computed t values are greater in magnitude.

[39] The fact that the results for PHYS are much weaker for states than for SMSA's is probably due to much higher correlations between PHYS and other independent variables in states.

[40] In the case of blacks the regression coefficients of CIG, in exploratory regressions, are positive and insignificant for males but negative and respectable for females. Given the crude nature of the black CIG estimates (see Appendix A), it was decided to exclude this variable from the black regressions. For reasons that are unclear the regression coefficient of CIG for white females is negative and insignificant when MS, PHYS, and FRTL are excluded (regression 1*). Charlotte Muller has suggested that race and sex differences in the effect of smoking might be due to differences in the time at which smoking became commonplace in the various groups.

pected negative sign and achieve statistical significance.[41] The elasticity of -0.05 for white females is relatively high.

TEMPERATURE (ATMP) AND SULFUR DIOXIDE AIR POLLUTION (SO₂D). The regressions for climate and air pollution variables are not presented in Table 9-3 because they differ somewhat in specification and because the relevant measures are unavailable for large numbers of SMSA's.[42] The results are summarized below.

The findings for average temperature (ATMP) are reasonably strong: (1) The regression coefficients are consistently negative and with the exception of black males achieve or approach statistical significance. (2) The inclusion of ATMP increases the adjusted coefficients of determination for each of the race-sex groups. That the coefficients of ATMP are negative suggests that, over the range considered, increases in average temperature reduce mortality rates.

The most promising of the available air pollution variables is SO₂D, but the results are mixed. While the coefficients of the dummy variable are usually *negative* but insignificant, the coefficients of the more sensitive rank variable always have the expected positive sign and are significant for whites.

Results for Two-Stage Least Squares

After some experimentation estimating equations were obtained for the endogenous variables. The coefficients of determination are shown in Table 9-2, while the second-stage equations are shown, with the ordinary least squares results, in Table 9-1. It should be noted that in order to satisfy the order condition for identifiability—i.e., "that the number of predetermined variables excluded from the relation must be at least as great as the number of endogenous variables included less one,"[43] it was necessary to exclude some exogenous variables from the SMSA regressions. The decision of which exogenous variables to exclude is not very difficult. First, REGN is sometimes excluded from the regressions for white females and is excluded from all the black female regressions because of extremely high correlations with total family income and its components (in the range of 0.9). Secondly, %RCC is excluded because it is not of the greatest interest and the ordinary least

---

[41] The male regression coefficients of WELF are also negative but they do not achieve significance. Since females are more likely to be strongly dependent upon public welfare payments than males, this result is not unreasonable, and it was considered appropriate to exclude WELF from the male regressions.

[42] Detailed tables are available from the author.

[43] Johnston, *Econometric Methods*, p. 251.

TABLE 9-2

Coefficients of Multiple Determination (R^2) for the First-Stage Natural Weighted Regressions for States and SMSA's

Endogenous Variables		White Males SMSA's (99 Observations)	White Males States (48 Observations)	White Females SMSA's (99 Observations)	White Females States (48 Observations)	Black Males SMSA's (59 Observations)	Black Males States (32 Observations)	Black Females SMSA's (99 Observations)	Black Females States (32 Observations)
MHWY	X_1	.564	.888	.492	.869	.220	.628	.842	.969
NLABY	X_{INL}	.606	.851	.511	.878	.794	.973	.788	.959
LABY	X_{IL}	.465	.854	.293	.757	.743	.976	.818	.959
MRTL	X_3	.606	.790	.588	.811	.821	.971	.614	.657
FRTL	X_4	.446	.764	.450	.767	.602	.914	.793	.977
MS	X_7	.359	.745	.433	.706	.840	.974	.822	.956
ULCR	X_{14}	.463		.298		.278		.494	
PHYS	X_{22}	.420	.835	.447	.829	.427	.896	.636	.893

Source: Available from the author on request.

squares findings are relatively weak and unstable. Assessments of the validity of the two-stage least squares results should take account of the fact that (a) the coefficients of determination for the first-stage regressions are sometimes quite low, which reduces the chances of obtaining significant regression coefficients for the endogenous variables, and (b) the simple correlations between some of the independent variables are quite high (above 0.8), which leads one to expect multicollinearity problems.[44]

With the exception of white females, where the evidence for a negative relationship between mortality and MHWY is sharply strengthened, the two-stage least squares results for income are like those for ordinary least squares. Turning to the other endogenous variables, the ordinary least squares results receive reasonably convincing support in the cases of schooling and the ulcer death rate, somewhat weaker support for marital status and physicians per capita, and little or none for fertility.

4. ANALYSIS OF RACE AND SEX DIFFERENTIALS IN MORTALITY RATES

In this section, the previous findings are applied to the problem of "explaining" race and sex differentials in age-adjusted mortality rates. After careful consideration of the preceding regressions it was decided to rely on three variants of the ordinary least squares regressions for SMSA's. In order to focus more clearly upon the role of income, variants I and II exclude the measures of schooling, fertility, and physicians per capita. Variant I utilizes total family income to measure command over goods and services. Variant II, however, represents an attempt to distinguish between the roles of labor and nonlabor income. In the case of white males, the coefficients of labor and nonlabor income are estimated separately, while for the other race-sex groups the coefficients of the latter variables are assumed to be equal to the estimated coefficients of total family income.[45] Variant III focuses on

---

[44] Such problems are, in fact, evidenced by sharp fluctuations in the coefficients and computed *t* values for some of the variables. In comparing the Auster, Leveson, and Sarachek results with those of this essay it should be remembered that they take income, schooling, the birth rate, and labor force participation rates for females to be *exogenous* variables.

[45] This procedure is considered appropriate because, in the regressions of Section 3, the white male coefficients of labor and nonlabor income not only differ sharply but behave in a stable and meaningful manner, which is not the case for the other race-sex groups.

the role of schooling and hence excludes the income measures as well as the measures of fertility and physicians per capita.

All variants differ from the regressions of Section 3 in that the white regressions are restricted to the fifty-nine SMSA's included in the black regressions in order to facilitate racial comparisons. The parameters of the regression equations are shown in Table 9-3.

The first step in the analysis is an over-all comparison between the mortality differentials predicted by each variant of the regression equation and the actual differentials. The procedure employed is as follows: The constant terms of the regression equations relevant for a given race or sex comparison are averaged, utilizing as weights the number in the appropriate race-sex groups (see Table 9-4); the appropriate values of the independent variable are then entered in the equations yielding predicted mortality rates for each SMSA; by subtraction, predicted mortality differentials are obtained for each SMSA; finally, the arithmetic mean of the predicted differentials is calculated and compared with the corresponding arithmetic mean of the actual, uncorrected[46] differentials. The constant terms are averaged in the first step because an observed difference in constant terms is unconvincing as an *explanation* of a race or sex mortality differential.

Line (2) of Table 9-5 reveals that the predicted and actual differentials being compared often have opposite signs (i.e., if the difference in the constant terms is put aside, the equations often predict that whites and females will have higher mortality rates than blacks and males). This finding may be indicative of substantive deficiencies in the specification of the equations, such as the omission or poor measurement of important independent variables. However, this is not necessarily the case. The predicted differentials are the result of differences between race-sex groups in *both* the levels and regression coefficients of the independent variables. It is of some interest to examine the differentials that can be attributed to differences in levels alone. First, the a priori arguments of Section 2 do not typically dictate differences in regression coefficients. Second, even though some differences in regression coefficients are significant, taken as a whole the formal tests must be regarded as inconclusive because of inconsistencies in the results.[47] In this connection it is well to remember that in certain

---

[46] It should be remembered that population underreporting is especially severe for blacks. The use of more accurate population figures, if available, might considerably reduce racial differentials in mortality rates.

[47] The tests are available upon request. The over-all inconsistency of the significance tests suggests the use of pooled regressions. Would the increase in

TABLE 9-3

Parameters of the Natural Weighted Variants I–III Regression Equations by Race-Sex Group for 59 SMSA's, 1959–61

Independent Variable		Variant I				Variant II	Variant III			
		WM	WF	BM	BF	WM	WM	WF	BM	BF
MHWY	X_1	−0.0000 (−0.35)	−0.0001 (−0.52)	−0.001 (−5.02)[b]	−0.0004 (−1.36)	—	—	—	—	—
NLABY	X_{1NL}	—	—	—	—	−0.001 (−3.64)[b]	—	—	—	—
LABY	X_{1L}	—	—	—	—	0.0003 (1.98)	—	—	—	—
MRTL	X_3	−0.084 (−3.82)[b]	−0.074 (−3.82)[b]	−0.196 (−4.09)[b]	−0.077 (−3.02)[b]	−0.122 (−5.56)[b]	−0.060 (−3.07)[b]	−0.047 (−3.19)[b]	−0.150 (−3.61)[b]	−0.050 (−2.56)[a]
REGN	X_5	—	−0.638 (−2.59)[a]	—	0.478 (1.01)	—	—	−0.473 (−3.43)[b]	—	−0.255 (−0.95)
MS	X_7	—	—	—	—	—	−0.312 (−4.21)[b]	−0.418 (−6.41)[b]	−0.838 (−6.61)[b]	−0.958 (−6.57)[b]

(continued)

TABLE 9-3 (concluded)

%RCC X₈	-0.020	0.235	2.590	1.568	0.119	-0.044	0.146	2.628	2.211
	(-0.05)	(0.64)	(2.01)ᵃ	(1.56)	(0.31)	(-0.12)	(0.54)	(2.30)ᵃ	(2.98)ᵇ
%BLK X₁₂	0.049	0.030	—	—	0.047	0.046	0.020	—	—
	(4.29)ᵇ	(2.53)ᵃ			(4.63)ᵇ	(4.74)ᵇ	(2.38)ᵃ		
ULCR X₁₄	0.078	0.190	0.102	0.138	0.117	0.096	0.168	0.103	0.120
	(1.46)	(1.77)	(2.03)ᵃ	(1.62)	(2.41)ᵃ	(2.40)ᵃ	(2.13)ᵃ	(2.27)ᵃ	(1.88)
Constant	16.07	11.46	26.32	14.21	18.33	17.47	14.18	26.39	19.76
R^2	0.415	0.543	0.419	0.341	0.544	0.561	0.754	0.529	0.624
$\bar{R}^2$	0.360	0.490	0.376	0.279	0.491	0.519	0.725	0.494	0.589

Note: The computed t values are in parentheses. The unweighted arithmetic mean values of the variables, by race-sex group, are as follows:

Variable		WM	WF	BM	BF
MHWY	X₁	6603.17	6603.17	4156.37	4156.37
NLABY	X₁NL	1822.27	5615.27	1228.01	3435.57
LABY	X₁L	4780.90	987.90	2932.69	725.12
MRTL	X₃	68.62	63.48	54.93	49.34
REGN	X₅	0.47	0.47	0.47	0.47
MS	X₇	11.16	11.37	8.31	9.08
%RCC	X₈	0.47	0.47	0.80	0.80
%BLK	X₁₂	14.30	14.30	14.30	14.30
ULCR	X₁₄	10.36	3.05	9.15	3.15

Source: Text.

ᵃ Indicates coefficient is significant at the .05 level of significance.

ᵇ Indicates coefficient is significant at the .01 level of significance.

TABLE 9-4

Weighted Averages of Parameters for the Variants I–III Regression Equations, by Race-Sex Groups, 59 SMSA's, 1959–61

		Variant I				Variant II		Variant III			
		Male	Female	White	Black	Male	White	Male	Female	White	Black
MHWY	X_1	-0.0001	-0.0001	-0.00005	-0.0007	-0.001	-0.0005	—	—	—	—
NLABY	X_{1NL}	—	—	—	—	0.0001	0.0001	—	—	—	—
LABY	X_{1L}	—	—	—	—	—	—	—	—	—	—
MRTL	X_3	-0.098	-0.075	-0.079	-0.134	-0.131	-0.098	-0.071	-0.047	-0.053	-0.098
REGN	X_5	—	-0.497	-0.327	0.250	—	-0.327	—	-0.446	-0.242	-0.134
MS	X_7	—	—	—	—	—	—	-0.376	-0.487	-0.367	-0.901
% RCC	X_8	0.298	0.404	0.111	2.055	0.420	0.179	0.281	0.407	0.053	2.410
% BLK	X_{12}	0.043	0.026	0.036	—	0.042	0.039	0.041	0.017	0.033	—
ULCR	X_{14}	0.081	0.184	0.136	0.121	0.116	0.155	0.097	0.162	0.133	0.111
Constant		17.32	11.81	13.71	19.98	19.30	14.81	18.56	14.89	15.78	22.92

Source: Table 9-3.

instances formal tests may, in effect, overstate the case of race and sex differentials. For example, differences in income coefficients might actually reflect the fact that black incomes are more strongly dependent upon health status than those of whites.[48] Finally, focusing on levels is desirable because even significant differences in parameters are often difficult to interpret and hence difficult to apply to policy problems. As an illustration, does an observed difference in regression coefficients reflect an intrinsic difference between the two race-sex groups being compared or does it merely reflect the fact that these groups differ in the level of the variable, with the coefficient varying systematically with level in both?

The procedure used to obtain predicted differentials attributable to differences in the levels of the independent variables is the same as that used for the over-all comparisons, with one major exception—the regression coefficients are averaged as well as the constant terms.[49] The results shown in lines (3) and (4) of Table 9-5 suggest the following conclusions.

1. The equations do quite well in explaining racial differentials in mortality rates. There is agreement between the signs of the mean predicted differentials and the signs of the mean actual differentials. The predicted differentials can be expressed as 31 per cent or more of the actual differentials. In conformity with the views of many students of this problem, income (or, alternatively, schooling) and the per cent married with spouse present are the variables whose level differences are most strongly associated with the excess of black over white mortality rates.

2. Utilizing variant II, mortality differentials predicted on the basis of differences in the levels of the independent variables represent

---

statistical efficiency resulting from a duplication of the analysis by means of pooled regressions justify the additional research effort? I think not, for the following reasons. First, there appear to be real race and sex differences in the constant terms, a consequence of which would be severe multicollinearity problems. Second, the technique used in the text is flexible enough to allow considering what seems to be a real sex difference in the regression coefficient of labor income. Finally, the technique utilized in the text produces results for race and sex differentials that are, generally speaking, strong and reasonable.

[48] I owe this point to William Landes.

[49] In this connection, when an independent variable is not included in the regression for one of the groups being compared, the regression coefficient is assumed to have a zero value. The predicted mortality rate that can be attributed to the level of a *given* independent variable is ascertained by inserting its values in the average equation while holding all other independent variables constant.

TABLE 9-5

Comparison of Arithmetic Mean Predicted and Actual Mortality Rate Differentials by Sex and Race Groups, SMSA's, 1959–61

Differentials (M-F or B-W)	Males			Females		Whites			Blacks	
	I	II	III	I	II	I	II	III	I	III
(1) Uncorrected mean actual differential	2.78	2.78	2.78	3.56	3.56	4.43	4.43	4.43	3.65	3.65
(2) Mean predicted differential due to levels and coefficients	−7.66	−5.13	−6.21	1.03	−2.07	0.29	−2.24	1.13	−8.40	−3.02
(3) Mean predicted differential due to levels	1.63	2.13	2.02	1.55	1.11	0.59	3.06	0.77	−0.02	0.82
as % of (1)	59	77	73	44	31	13	69	17	−0.5	22
(4) Mean predicted differential due to levels of individual variables:										
MHWY (X_1)	0.29	—	—	0.34	—	—	—	—	—	—
as % of (1)	10			10						
NLABY (X_{1NL})	—	0.60	—	—	—	—	2.05	—	—	—
as % of (1)		22					46			
LABY (X_{1L})	−0.26	—	—	—	—	—	0.38	—	—	—
as % of (1)	−9						9			
MRTL (X_3)	1.34	1.79	0.97	1.06	0.67	−0.41	−0.50	−0.27	−0.75	−0.55
as % of (1)	48	64	35	30	19	−9	−11	−6	−20	−16
MS (X_7)	—	—	1.07	—	1.11	—	—	0.08	—	0.70
as % of (1)			39		31			2		19
% RCC (X_8)	0.10	0.14	0.09	0.13	0.13	—	—	—	—	—
as % of (1)	3	5	3	4	4					
ULCR (X_{14})	−0.10	−0.14	−0.12	0.02	0.02	0.99	1.13	0.97	0.73	0.67
as % of (1)	−4	−5	−4	0.5	0.5	22	26	22	20	18

Source: Text and Table 9-4.

about 70 per cent of the excess of white male over white female mortality rates. The key differences in levels are that the ulcer death rate (a measure of psychological tension) is higher for males than for females,[50] while the ratio of nonlabor to total family income is higher for females than for males.

3. Utilizing variant III, differentials predicted on the basis of differences in the levels of the independent variables represent 24 per cent of the excess of black male over black female mortality rates. The key differences are that black females have more schooling than black males and that, as in the case of whites, females have lower ulcer death rates than males.

5. SUMMARY OF MAIN FINDINGS AND SUGGESTIONS FOR FUTURE RESEARCH

The most interesting and important findings, based on regressions run across states and standard metropolitan statistical areas, with age-adjusted mortality as the dependent variable, are listed below.

1. In multiple regressions excluding schooling, the coefficients of family income are typically negative. This relationship is much stronger for black than for white males and is much more evident across SMSA's than across states. For white males across states the relationship is positive.

2. When family income is crudely decomposed into labor and nonlabor components, the results suggest that for white males the observed coefficient of family income represents a compromise between the favorable health effects of a "pure" increase in income and the unfavorable (or less favorable) health effects of increases in earnings. When the total family income of white males is replaced by their nonlabor income, the observed racial differential in income effects is considerably narrowed.

3. The ordinary least-squares regression coefficients for schooling are strongly negative and usually achieve statistical significance.

4. An inverse relationship that seems especially strong for black males is observed between the mortality rate and the per cent married with spouse present.

5. The mortality rate is positively correlated with a measure of psychological tension (the death rate from ulcers of the stomach).

[50] The psychological tension interpretation would have to be modified in the case of the sex differences to the extent that the male-female differential in susceptibility to ulcers is due to physiological (hormonal) differences.

6. Nontrivial shares of the excess of black over white mortality rates can be attributed to differences in income (or schooling) levels and, even more importantly, in percentages married with spouse present.

7. The ratio of nonlabor to total family income may account for a major share of the excess of white male over white female mortality. Differences in the ulcer death rate also work in this direction.

8. The excess of black male over black female mortality may be related to the greater schooling of black females. Sex differences in ulcer death rates are also noted.

Meanwhile, the limitations of the study must be kept in mind, notably the following: (1) The regression analysis is confined to spatial (or "ecological") data for the period 1959–61. Lagged values of the independent variables are not included in the regressions and results are not checked by means of time series data or data for individuals. (2) Health is measured by age-adjusted mortality rates for all ages. Alternative measures of health (e.g., "disability days") are not considered and little or no attention is paid to age-specific and specific-cause mortality rates. One of the major conclusions of Appendix B is that the "probability" is quite low (0.28 to 0.49) that a geographic unit having a high mortality rate for one age group will have relatively high rates for other age groups. (3) Attempts to increase knowledge concerning the health effects of air pollution are seriously hampered by the use of published pollution data which are expressed only in rank form. (4) Collinearity problems make it difficult to disentangle the effects of certain variables (most importantly, family income versus schooling or the earnings rate). (5) The income measures employed in the study are undeflated, which, according to pilot regressions, imparts a bias to the income coefficients. (6) The regression analysis does not include direct measures of the relative prices of medical care and other health-producing (or health-inhibiting) goods and services. There is great need for such price measures.

There is also need for new studies utilizing different methodologies and types of data. In my opinion, first priority should be given to further study of the roles of income, schooling, and marital status. The latter variables appear to be crucial in explaining the excess of black over white mortality, but the exact causal mechanisms are still uncertain.

We need more definitive answers to a number of questions. For example, "pure" increases in income are spent in ways that improve health status, but exactly which purchased goods and services are primarily responsible? How important is medical care as compared to health-related items like proper nutrition and adequate recreation?

Exactly which labor force activities are responsible for the observed positive correlation between earnings and the mortality rate of white males? To what extent should the observed beneficial health effects of schooling be attributed to an increased use of medical services? How important is training in such topics as personal hygiene and nutrition? Should increased use of medical and health-related goods and services be attributed to the fact that persons with more schooling know better how to seek out and select the appropriate items? Or does schooling, perhaps, reflect or increase the "taste" for good health and consequently the demand? Is it the real answer that schooling is an excellent proxy for wealth and certain occupational factors and has little or no independent effect upon health? Which of the possible lines of explanation of the role of marital status is most relevant—that married persons place a higher relative value on their health than single persons or that being married lowers the relative prices of a number of health-producing items? Until we have the answers to these related questions both policy and theory will suffer.

APPENDIX A: DETAILS ON VARIABLES INCLUDED IN THE REGRESSION ANALYSIS[51]

Y (**DDR**): See Edward A. Duffy and Robert E. Carroll, *United States Metropolitan Mortality, 1959–61,* U.S. Department of Health, Education, and Welfare, Public Health Service, Cincinnati, Bureau of Disease Prevention and Environmental Control, 1967, Table 4.

Age adjustment is by the direct method (see note to Table 9–B-4).

Y′ (**IDR**): See note to Table 9–B-1 and footnote 53.

X_1 (**MHWY**): See *Census of Population, 1960,* State Tables 133 and 139 and National Summary Table 224.

In the 1960 census, "total income" is the sum of wage and salary income, self-employment income, and other income. "Other income" includes net receipts from rents, royalties, interest, dividends, periodic income from estates and trust funds, social security benefits, pensions,

---

[51] See definitions of all variables included in the regressions on pp. 163–166.

veterans payments, military allotments for dependents, unemployment insurance, public assistance or other governmental payments, periodic contributions from persons who are not members of the household, alimony, and periodic receipts from insurance policies or annuities. The figures represent the amount of income received before deductions for personal income taxes, social security, bond purchases, union dues, et cetera. Not included as income are the following: money received from the sale of property; the value of income "in kind," such as food produced or consumed in the home or free living quarters; withdrawals of bank deposits; money borrowed; tax refunds; gifts and lump-sum inheritance or insurance benefits. Measures of median income are readily available in the census data and the median has the advantage of holding transitory components to a minimum.

X'_1 (**MPY**): See source for X_1.

X'''_1 (%**LT3T**): See source for X_1.

The percentage of husband-wife families in each age group with annual cash incomes of less than $3,000 (using this as the "poverty line") is computed and then averaged, with the national percentage of husband-wife families in each age group used as weights.

X_{1L} (**LABY**): See source for X_1 and *Census of Population, 1960,* State Table 144.

In accordance with a decision to focus attention on sources of the income of the head of the family or his wife, (a) the estimate of the labor component of income for a given race-sex group is the median annual earnings of that group (for persons with earnings) multiplied, in the case of males, by the fraction of husband-wife families in which the head worked in 1959 and, in the case of females, by the fraction in which the wife worked in 1959 (X_{1L}); and (b) the estimate of nonlabor income (X_{1NL}) for a given race-sex group is obtained as a residual by subtracting X_{1L} of the sex group whose mortality is being studied from the MHWY (X_1) of the corresponding race group—e.g., the nonlabor income of white females is obtained by subtracting the median (weighted) earnings of white females from white husband-wife income.

X_{1NL} **(NLABY)**: See notes for X_1, X_2, and LABY.

X_2 **(EARNR)**: *Census of Population, 1960,* State Tables 124 and 118.

Weekly earnings rates are obtained by dividing median annual earnings for persons with earnings in 1959 by the median number of weeks worked by those working in that year. In general, the weekly earnings rate resulting from the above division will not be equal to the (unavailable) median weekly earnings rate of the individuals in an area. However, while random errors in an independent variable cause underestimates of the regression coefficient, I can see no reason for believing that our proxy measure will be systematically biased.

X_3 **(MRTL)**: *Census of Population, 1960,* State Tables 109 and 96 and National Summary Table 46.

The number of husband-wife families in each group is used as the number of married males or females. The percentage married in each age group is obtained by dividing the above numbers by the number of males or females in each age group (fourteen to twenty-four was used for the youngest age group). The national percentages of those age fourteen and over in each age group are used as weights.

X_4 **(FRTL)**: *Census of Population, 1960,* State Table 113 and National Summary Table 190.

The children-ever-born measure is superior to the birth rate, which might be considered an index of the rationality of current behavior, because current health is dependent not only on present behavior but on the extent to which past decisions were rational.

X_6 **(FB)**: *Census of Population, 1960,* State Table 96.

X_7 **(MS)**: *Census of Population, 1960,* State Table 103.

X_8 **(%RC)**: *Census of Population, 1960,* State Tables 14 and 15, Final Report.

Pc (3)–10, Selected Area Reports, *Standard Metropolitan Statistical Areas,* Table 1.

X'_8 **(RUA)** : See sources for X_8.

X_9 **(%LAB)**: *Census of Population, 1960,* State Table 122.

X_{10} **(%MWLFPC)**: *Census of Population, 1960,* State Table 116.

X_{11} **(%MFG)**: *Census of Population, 1960,* State Table 129.

X_{12} **(%BLK)**: *Census of Population, 1960,* State Table 90.

X_{13} **(SEG)**: Wendell Bell and Ernest W. Willis, "The Segregation of Negroes in American Cities: A Comparative Analysis," *Social and Economic Studies,* March 1957, Appendix.

X_{13} is based upon data for census tracts: if the percentage of blacks residing on a block is equal to the percentage of blacks in the tract, the index takes a value of 0; at the other extreme, if the percentage of blacks residing on the block is 0 or 100, the index takes the value of 100.

X_{14} **(ULCR)** : See source for *Y.*

X'_{14} **(ULCRD)** : See source for *Y.*

X_{15} **(ATMP)**, X_{16} **(AHUM)**, X_{17} **(DTMP)**, X_{18} **(DHUM)** : U.S. Department of Commerce, Weather Bureau, Environmental Services Administration, *Climatological Data: National Summary for 1960, 1961.*

The data are averages for weather stations in the standard metropolitan statistical area. X_{18} is based upon relative humidity measures for 1 A.M. and 1 P.M., E.S.T.

X_{19} **(GASDR)**, X_{20} **(ACSPR)**, X_{21} **(SO_2DR)**: U.S. Department of Health, Education, and Welfare, Public Health Service, National Center for Air Pollution Control, HEW-R43, August 4, 1967.

X_{22} **(PHYS)**: *Census of Population, 1960,* State Tables 120 and 133.

X_{23} **(%HOUS)**: *U.S. Census of Housing, 1960,* U.S. Summary, States and Small Areas, Tables 6 and 25 and Series $HC(_1)$, States and Small Areas, Tables 15, 37, 38.
The housing data are for owner-occupied and renter-occupied rooms.

X_{24} **(POPD)**: U.S. Department of Commerce, Bureau of the Census, *County and City Data Book: 1962,* Table 1, item 4 and Table 3, item 4.

X_{25} **(%FS)**: *Census of Population, 1960,* State Table 100.

X_{26} **(CIG)**: *Tobacco Smoking Patterns in the United States,* Public Health Monograph No. 45, 1956, Tables 146 and 15a.
The underlying data are percentages of persons age eighteen and over in two smoking categories: ½ to 1 and 1 or more packs of cigarettes per day. The percentages are cross-classified by region, sex, residence (urban, rural nonfarm, and rural farm), and, in the South, by race (white or nonwhite). For Southern states the percentage of a sex-race-residence group in a given smoking category is estimated by the corresponding percentage for the entire region, and for each state the percentage of a sex-race group in a given smoking category is obtained by averaging the appropriate regional percentages using as weights the state's 1960 residence distribution of the race-sex group. Next, the estimated fractions for a state are divided by the correspond-

ing percentages for the entire United States (both races and sexes). Finally, the indexes for the ½–1 and 1 or more pack smoking categories are averaged, with the 1 or more pack category receiving twice the weight of the ½–1 pack category. The procedure for non-Southern states is the same as for the Southern states, with the exception that, since a race breakdown is not available for each of the non-Southern regions, it is assumed that the percentage of a sex-residence group in a given smoking category does not vary with race. Available data for the North and West combined reveal some sharp differences in the cigarette consumption of whites and nonwhites, but nonwhites who reside outside the South are concentrated in urban areas, and in such areas color differences in consumption are fairly small. For the ½ to 1 pack category, the ratio of the percentage for white males to that for nonwhite males is 0.85, while that for the 1 or more pack category is 1.63; the corresponding values for females are 1.09 and 0.97.

X_{27} **(WTRH):** Henry A. Schroeder, "Relation Between Mortality from Cardiovascular Disease and Treated Water Supplies," *Journal of the American Medical Association,* 172, April 23, 1960, pp. 1902–08, Table 1.

X_{27} is obtained by weighting the average hardness of each type of water supply (surface or ground) by the population served by that supply; the data refer to 1950–51.

X_{28} **(HIGHW),** X_{29} **(WELF),** X_{30} **(HOSP),** X_{31} **(HLTH),** X_{32} **(POL),** X_{33} **(FIRE),** X_{34} **(SAN):** U.S. Department of Commerce, *Census of Government, 1962,* IV, Table 37.

Total public welfare includes support of and assistance to needy persons contingent on their need. Excluded are pensions to former employees and other benefits not contingent on need. Expenditures include: (a) cash assistance payments made directly to needy persons under categorical and other welfare programs; (b) vendor payments made to private purveyors for medical care, burials, and other services provided under welfare programs; (c) welfare institutions (includes other unspecified items and intergovernmental expenditures). Any services provided directly by the government through its own *Hospitals* and *Health* agencies are classed under those headings.

Supplementary Variables

X'_8 (%RUA) : *Census of Population, 1960,* State Tables 14 and 15.

X_{24N} (TPOP) : U.S. Bureau of the Census, *Statistical Abstract of the United States, 1969,* Section 33, Table 1 and Section 1, Table 13.

X_{28} (UO) : Leo Troy, *Distribution of Union Membership Among the States, 1939 and 1953,* New York, NBER, 1957, p. 18, Table 4.

X_{29} (RS) : Calculated from data in Lowell D. Ashby, "The Geographical Redistribution of Employment," *Survey of Current Business,* October 1964, p. 15, Table 3.

X_{29} depends on whether rate of growth of each state's industry was rapid or slow compared with the national growth rates of these industries.

APPENDIX B: A DESCRIPTIVE ANALYSIS OF MORTALITY RATES FOR CENSUS DIVISIONS[52]

Purpose and Main Conclusions

The objective of this appendix is to ascertain the magnitudes and patterns of spatial differences in mortality and to make comparisons of such differences by race and sex. The analysis is designed to provide a useful background for the multivariate analysis of mortality rates presented in the text and to suggest new hypotheses or questions. The data employed are for the nine geographic divisions of the United States in 1959–61. Data for census divisions should make apparent any interesting spatial patterns without burdening the reader with excessive detail. Generally, when measures of association are needed both Spearman rank and product-moment correlation coefficients (unweighted) are utilized. For present purposes, the major advantage of the coefficient of rank correlation is that it reduces the weight given to extreme observations, which can be important when the number of observations is small (as in the present case) or when relationships are nonlinear. Mortality data for all ages are examined in the second part of this appendix; age-specific mortality rates are explored in the third part.

[52] I wish to thank Mortimer Spiegelman for his helpful comments on an earlier draft of this appendix.

The major findings of the descriptive analysis are as follows:

1. When attention is shifted from unadjusted mortality rates to age- and sex-adjusted mortality ratios, it becomes evident that the black rates are substantially higher than their white counterparts in every census division.

2. Age and sex adjustments sharply alter spatial patterns in mortality rates. The simple correlations between the unadjusted and adjusted rates are only 0.61 for whites and 0.34 for blacks.

3. Age and sex adjustments substantially reduce the magnitudes of spatial variations in mortality—from 10.2 to 4.1 per cent for whites and from 14.0 to 5.6 per cent for blacks. In the case of whites, the female coefficient of variation exceeds the male coefficient, and variability is smallest in the fifteen–sixty-four age group. Just the opposite is true for nonwhites.

4. For both races, age-adjusted mortality rates are higher for males than for females in every census division; spatial patterns are quite similar for males and females—the simple correlations are 0.84 for whites and 0.79 for blacks. These high correlations result from strong relationships in the under-fifteen and sixty-five-and-over age group.

5. Of interest in reference to the possible "reversal" of socioeconomic male-female roles within the black subculture is the fact that the spatial pattern of mortality rates for black females resembles that of white males as much as or more strongly than it resembles the pattern for white females.

6. Year-to-year variation in mortality rates for 1959–61 is not large for any census division, but spatial variability in the amount of year-to-year variation is appreciable. The latter type of variation is greater for females and blacks than for males and whites. Evidence of racial differences within divisions in the character of the forces determining year-to-year variability is provided by rather low correlations between the divisional measures of year-to-year variation.

7. There exists, especially in the case of females, an inverse relationship between levels and year-to-year variability in mortality.

8. The probability that a census division having a high mortality rate for one age group will have relatively high rates for the other ages is somewhat higher for females and nonwhites than for males and whites. However, the probabilities are quite low, ranging from 0.28 to 0.49.

Analysis of Mortality Data for All Ages

Table 9—B-1 is designed to facilitate comparisons of spatial levels and

TABLE 9–B–1

Unadjusted and Age- and Sex-adjusted Mortality Rates by Race
for U.S. Census Divisions in the Period 1959–61

Census Division	Whites		Blacks	
	Deaths per 1,000 Population	Age- and Sex-adjusted Mortality Ratio	Deaths per 1,000 Population	Age- and Sex-adjusted Mortality Ratio
Northeast	10.54	0.99	9.01	1.38
Middle Atlantic	10.54	1.03	9.82	1.48
East North Central	9.54	0.98	9.20	1.40
West North Central	9.92	0.90	11.90	1.39
South Atlantic	8.37	0.94	10.53	1.51
East South Central	8.73	0.95	11.54	1.36
West South Central	8.16	0.91	10.50	1.26
Mountain	7.95	0.95	9.12	1.40
Pacific	8.84	0.93	7.18	1.23
Coefficient of variation (%)	10.21	4.13	13.83	6.16
Percentage point differential in coefficients of variation	6.08		7.67	
Percentage reduction in coefficient of variation	84.80		76.74	
Rank coefficient of correlation	0.42		0.23	
Product moment coefficient of correlation	0.61		0.34	

Note: Age-sex adjusted by the "indirect" method. For each state, 1959–61 national (excluding Alaska, Hawaii, and Washington, D.C.) age-specific death rates for whites and blacks, both sexes combined, were multiplied by the actual population distributions by race and sex in 1960 to obtain "expected" deaths. The "expected" deaths of males and females of a given race were summed and the result was divided into the sum of the actual deaths to obtain a mortality ratio, i.e., the age- and sex-adjusted death rate in index number form (U.S. whites and blacks equal 1). By using national age-specific rates for both races and sexes as a single standard it is possible to make comparisons of levels of mortality among sexes and races as well as geographic areas.

Sources: *Mortality:* U.S. Department of Health, Education and Welfare, Public Health Service, National Vital Statistics Division, *Vital Statistics of the United States*, 1959—Tables 62 and 71, 1960 and 1961—Tables 5-4 and 5-9. *Population:* U.S. Bureau of the Census, *Census of Population*, 1960, Volume I, Characteristics of the Population, Part 1, United States Summary, Table 158 and Parts 2–52 (State Volumes), Table 96.

variations in the unadjusted and age- and sex-adjusted[53] mortality rates of whites and blacks. Perhaps the most striking fact exhibited by the table is that once we turn from unadjusted to adjusted mortality rates the black rate is substantially higher than the white in every division.[54] Turning to detailed comparisons of the adjusted and unadjusted data, it is observed that for whites the unadjusted rates for Northern divisions, especially the Northeast and Middle Atlantic, are relatively high. In the adjusted data, the Northern disadvantage is retained but is clearly reduced, while the rates for Southern and Western divisions remain quite similar. For blacks the unadjusted rates are especially high in the Southern divisions and low in the Pacific division. However, with age and sex adjustments, the Southern rates are found not to differ greatly from Northern ones and the Pacific advantage is substantially reduced. That age and sex adjustment significantly alters spatial patterns in mortality is most conveniently summarized by the relatively low correlations between the adjusted and unadjusted mortality rates. For whites the product-moment correlation is 0.61 and the rank correlation is 0.42, while the corresponding values for blacks are 0.34 and 0.23.

Age and sex adjustment also reduces substantially the magnitude of spatial variation in mortality—from 10.2 to 4.1 per cent for whites and from 14.0 to 5.6 per cent for blacks. It is worth noting that in relative terms the mortality of blacks varies substantially more than that of whites. The residual variation in mortality is not very large for either race, but it is believed to be large enough to make the more formal analysis presented in the text meaningful.

[53] Mortality is adjusted by the "indirect" method, the major advantage of which is that, unlike "direct" standardization, it does not require the allocation of scarce research resources to the tabulation of age-specific mortality rates by race and sex for each geographic unit. A defect of the indirect technique is that differences among geographic units (or races or sexes) are affected by differences in age distributions, unless the ratios of the (unknown) age-specific mortality rates for the geographic units (or races or sexes) being compared are invariant with respect to age. In this connection it should be noted that differences in directly standardized mortality rates are sensitive to changes in the standard population utilized. For details of the indirect age-sex adjustment, see note to Table 9–B–1.

[54] The relative underenumeration of the black population does not explain these differentials. According to Siegel, if there were no underregistration of deaths, and "if corrected population data are employed, life expectancy of nonwhites at birth in 1959–61 would be increased by about 1-1/2 years and most of the large white-nonwhite difference would remain" (J. Siegel, "Completeness of Coverage of the Nonwhite Population," 1968, p. 24).

Table 9–B-2 presents age-adjusted[55] mortality rates by sex, permitting a more refined analysis of spatial levels and patterns than is possible in Table 9–B-1. It is seen that for each race the male mortality rate is higher than the female one within each geographic division.[56] As expected, the patterns of spatial variation are very similar to those observed in Table 9–B-1. For whites of each sex the Northeast and Middle Atlantic are relatively high and the West South Central is relatively low, while the rates for the other divisions do not differ appreciably; for blacks the rates for the Middle Atlantic and South Atlantic are relatively high, while the Pacific rate is relatively low, especially in the case of females. The similarity of the spatial patterns for males and females is indicated by rather high coefficients of correlation: for whites the product-moment correlation is 0.84 and the rank correlation is 0.88, while for blacks the values are 0.79 and 0.72. However, it is clear from these coefficients that there are nontrivial sex differences in mortality patterns.

Turning to comparisons by race, the evidence lends some credence to current discussions suggesting the existence of a "reversal" of the socioeconomic roles of males and females within the black subculture. First, while the spatial patterns for white and black males are reasonably similar (the product-moment correlation is 0.62 and the rank correlation is 0.65), there is much less similarity between the patterns for females (the product-moment correlation is 0.39 and the rank correlation is 0.30). More significant for the reversal of roles argument is the fact that the spatial pattern for the black females resembles that of the white males about as much or more strongly (the product-moment correlation is 0.35, while the rank correlation is 0.53) than it resembles the pattern for white females. Along the same line, the correlations between black males and white females are surprisingly high (0.56 for the product-moment method and 0.45 for the rank correlation). Another point to be noted is the striking race difference in the relative magnitudes of spatial variations in mortality. For whites the female coefficient of variation is much higher than the very low male coefficient, while for blacks the male coefficient of variation is somewhat higher than that for females.

---

[55] For details of the method of age adjustment, see note to Table 9–B-2.

[56] The male population is subject to greater underenumeration than the female population (see Siegel, "Completeness of Coverage"), but it is unlikely that sex differentials in the accuracy of enumeration would completely explain the observed sex differentials in mortality.

TABLE 9–B–2

Age-adjusted Mortality Ratios for Males and Females by Race
for U.S. Census Divisions in the Period 1959–61

Census Division	Whites		Blacks	
	Age-adjusted Mortality Ratio for Males	Age-adjusted Mortality Ratio for Females	Age-adjusted Mortality Ratio for Males	Age-adjusted Mortality Ratio for Females
Northeast	1.23	0.81	1.64	1.15
Middle Atlantic	1.27	0.84	1.78	1.23
East North Central	1.20	0.79	1.62	1.20
West North Central	1.12	0.72	1.60	1.19
South Atlantic	1.20	0.72	1.79	1.27
East South Central	1.19	0.74	1.55	1.19
West South Central	1.16	0.69	1.45	1.08
Mountain	1.18	0.73	1.66	1.13
Pacific	1.17	0.72	1.49	1.01
Coefficient of variation (%)	3.38	6.17	6.80	6.41
Percentage point differential in coefficients of variation (male minus female)	−2.79		0.39	
Percentage of difference in coefficients of variation	−58.43		5.74	

Summary of Mortality Rate Correlations

Race-Sex Group	Rank Correlation Coefficient	Product-Moment Correlation Coefficient
White male-white female	.88	.84
Negro male-Negro female	.72	.79
White male-Negro male	.65	.62
White female-Negro female	.30	.39
White male-Negro female	.53	.35
White female-Negro male	.45	.56

Note: Age adjustment is by the "indirect" method. For each state, 1959–61 national (excluding Alaska, Hawaii, and Washington D.C.) age-specific death rates for whites and Negroes of both sexes combined were multiplied by the actual population distributions by race and sex in 1960 to obtain "expected" deaths. The "expected" deaths for a given race and sex were divided into the corresponding number of actual deaths to obtain a mortality ratio, i.e., the age-adjusted death rate in index number form (U.S. whites and Negroes equals 1). By using national age-specific rates for both races and sexes as a single standard it is possible to make comparisons of levels of mortality among races and sexes as well as geographically.

Source: See Table 9–B–1.

TABLE 9–B-3

Year-to-Year Variability in Deaths by Sex and Race

for U.S. Census Divisions in the Period 1959–61

(coefficients of variation of deaths, per cent)

	Whites			Blacks		
	Total	Male	Female	Total	Male	Female
Northeast	1.07	1.51	0.71	1.65	1.64	2.05
Middle Atlantic	0.64	0.84	0.45	3.20	3.47	2.90
East North Central	0.77	0.75	0.80	1.84	2.21	1.40
West North Central	1.21	0.83	1.76	0.28	0.76	0.70
South Atlantic	2.64	2.56	2.80	1.91	2.27	1.59
East South Central	1.80	1.93	1.77	1.96	2.28	1.63
West South Central	2.11	2.15	2.06	2.47	2.46	2.52
Mountain	1.55	1.31	1.96	1.26	2.77	4.95
Pacific	2.13	1.90	2.44	4.57	5.08	3.89
Coefficient of variation	41.5	39.9	46.6	53.8	44.6	52.3

Summary of Coefficient of Variation Correlations

Race-Sex Group	Rank Correlation Coefficient	Product-Moment Correlation Coefficient
White male-white female	.72	.74
Black male-black female	.85	.69
White male-black male	.25	.21
White female-black female	.15	.16
White male-black female	.20	.08
White female-black male	.28	.20

Source: See Table 9–B-1.

Table 9–B-3 provides information on the stability of mortality within the various geographic sex-race cells during the period with which we are concerned (1959–61), and also permits comparison of stability according to the previously utilized principles of classification. It should be noted that year-to-year variability is not very great; the highest coefficient of variation is 5.1 (for black males in the Pacific) and most of the values in the table are substantially lower than this. However, when we turn to spatial variability in the amount of year-to-year variation, it is observed that for both sexes and races it is substantial—in the range of 40–50 per cent. Clearly, the factors responsible for year-to-year variability in mortality are more constant within than among census divisions.

Among blacks there is a tendency for year-to-year variability to be greater for males than for females; this tendency also appears among whites but in a much weaker form. By contrast, for both races the spatial variability in the coefficients of variation is greater among females than males. It seems that males are more susceptible to year-to-year changes in the forces influencing mortality, but that spatially they have more in common with respect to these forces than females. An explanation might be based on the fact that males play a greater and more spatially constant role in the economy than females and are more strongly affected by fluctuations in business conditions. While substantial variation remains "unexplained," the patterns of spatial variability are similar for males and females of a given race: for whites the product-moment correlation is 0.74 and the rank correlation, 0.72, and for blacks the corresponding values are 0.69 and 0.85.

Levels of year-to-year variability are greater for blacks than for whites, with the exception of the West North Central, South Atlantic, and East South Central divisions. In addition, the spatial variability in the divisional coefficients of variation is greater for blacks than for whites. In view of factors like greater reporting errors for blacks and their greater susceptibility to infectious diseases, it is not surprising that black mortality should vary more than white. However, the basis for the exceptions noted above is not apparent.

The coefficients of correlation between the divisional coefficients of variation are quite low. The product-moment correlation for males is 0.21 and the rank correlation is 0.25, while the corresponding values for females are 0.16 and 0.15. Obviously, there are sharp racial differences within divisions in the character of the forces determining year-to-year variability in mortality. Again there is some evidence of a reversal of the male-female roles among blacks. In terms of the spatial pattern in year-to-year variability, black males are as much or more closely related to white females (the product-moment correlation is 0.20 and the rank correlation is 0.28) than they are to white males; and according to the rank correlations, black females are more closely related to white males (0.20) than they are to white females. However, the above conclusion is weakened by the fact that the product-moment correlation between white males and black females is only 0.08.

The data presented in Tables 9–B-2 and 9–B-3 hint that there may exist a positive relationship between the level of mortality and the magnitude of year-to-year variability. For a given sex, black age-adjusted mortality rates are always higher than white rates and there is also a tendency for their levels of year-to-year variability to be greater; for a given race, female age-adjusted mortality rates are always lower than male rates and there is a weak tendency for their levels of year-to-year variability to be lower. A possible explanation for the black-white finding is that, since the white population is larger, its mortality is less subject to random variations (including measurement errors) than black mortality.

In order to obtain better evidence bearing on the existence of such a relationship, product-moment correlations between divisional age-adjusted mortality rates and coefficients of year-to-year variations were run for each race-sex group. The coefficients are as follows: -0.13 for white males, -0.87 for white females, -0.15 for black males, and -0.57 for black females. Thus, the more refined evidence suggests, especially for females, an *inverse* relationship between levels and year-to-year variability in mortality. It would seem that the under-lying factors distinguishing relatively high and low mortality areas are rather stable, at least over periods as short as three years. A possible example of such a factor might be high birth rates and the associated large family sizes, which raise female mortality rates, directly or indirectly.

Analysis of Mortality Data by Age

In an attempt to obtain new insights concerning the magnitudes and patterns of spatial differences in mortality, data for census divisions were broken down according to age. In the interest of clarity—and to restrict our problem to manageable proportions—a limited number of meaningful and readily available age categories are employed: under fifteen, fifteen–sixty-four, and sixty-five and over. Because of the unavailability of black age-adjusted mortality rates by age, reliance is placed upon data for nonwhites adjusted by the direct method.[57] The rates are explored in Table 9–B-4. First, it is evident that within each

[57] The evidence presented in the note to Table 9–B-4 indicates that (1) there are nontrivial differences in the spatial mortality patterns of blacks and nonwhites (this is probably because the rates for nonwhites in the Mountain States are influenced by Indians and those on the Pacific Coast by Orientals) and (2) patterns may differ appreciably according to the method of age-adjustment. Nevertheless, it is felt that the data utilized in this appendix are adequate for its limited purposes. In the text, the use of nonwhite data is restricted to states and SMSA's in which nonwhites are overwhelmingly blacks and the multivariate analysis utilizes both directly and indirectly standardized mortality ratios.

TABLE 9–B–4

Age-adjusted Mortality Rates for Three Age Groups by Sex and Color
for U.S. Census Divisions in the Period 1959–61

	White Males			White Females		
Census Division	Persons Under 15 Years Old	Persons Age 15–64	Persons Age 65 and Over	Persons Under 15 Years Old	Persons Age 15–64	Persons Age 65 and Over
N.E.	216.5	553.4	7141.2	158.7	284.0	4908.8
M.A.	212.3	571.7	7349.6	158.8	303.8	5225.3
E.N.C.	218.7	548.8	7001.0	161.8	281.8	4826.6
W.N.C.	218.5	508.8	6392.3	158.6	246.0	4311.3
S.A.	238.2	601.7	6514.4	172.7	265.5	4395.8
E.S.C.	243.9	579.9	6493.2	193.9	257.4	4504.6
W.S.C.	246.4	555.1	6385.6	184.8	248.1	4079.6
M.	262.6	576.6	6417.0	191.9	281.3	4234.0
P.	225.3	557.1	6592.5	165.7	279.5	4264.5
Coefficient of variation (%)	6.99	4.34	5.15	8.03	6.60	7.87
Coefficient of concordance		0.28			0.32	

(continued)

age-race group the male mortality rate is higher than the female,[58] while in a number of census divisions the nonwhite mortality rate for a given age-sex group, with the exception of the sixty-five and over age group, is higher than the white.[59]

[58] See footnote 54.

[59] The fact that blacks in the older groups have lower mortality rates than whites is well known and is usually explained by the exceptional health characteristics of those blacks able to attain old age and discrepancies in population age reporting for blacks. For discussions of these issues, see Robert D. Grove, "Vital Statistics for the Negro, Puerto Rican, and Mexican Population: Present Quality and Plans for Improvement," *Social Statistics and the City,* a report of a conference sponsored by the Joint Center for Urban Studies of the Massachusetts Institute of Technology and Harvard University (held in Washington, D.C., June 22–23, 1967), Cambridge, Mass., 1968; and Melvin Zelnik, "Age Patterns of Mortality of American Negroes: 1900–02 to 1959–61," *Journal of the American Statistical Association,* 64, June 1969, pp. 443–51. Zelnik concludes (p. 446): "It appears to be quite likely, if not certain, that the low rates of mortality recorded in the official life tables for Negroes above age sixty-five are the result of age misreporting, which thereby also spuriously heightens somewhat the rates of mortality in the immediately prior age groups. However, the bulk of the available evidence suggests that the difference is real

TABLE 9-B-4 (continued)

Nonwhite Males			Nonwhite Females		
Persons Under 15 Years Old	Persons Age 15–64	Persons Age 65 and Over	Persons Under 15 Years Old	Persons Age 15–64	Persons Age 65 and Over
365.0	780.6	7368.7	268.7	540.9	5373.7
427.0	944.8	7036.1	328.6	633.3	5233.5
365.5	855.1	6980.4	291.0	648.4	5222.6
408.0	935.1	7134.0	332.3	678.5	5320.4
450.7	1099.6	6746.6	351.3	783.6	4911.6
443.8	939.3	6763.8	355.7	713.7	5226.7
410.4	866.9	6207.2	330.4	651.8	4596.2
502.7	876.3	5438.1	406.9	564.9	4230.1
313.4	587.1	5739.5	238.8	409.8	4171.7
12.87	14.99	9.45	14.66	16.35	9.06
	0.44			0.49	

Summary of Mortality Rate Correlations

Color-Sex Groups	Age	Rank Correlation Coefficient	Product-Moment Correlation Coefficient
White male-white female	Under 15	.88	.94
White male-white female	15–64	.05	.30
White male-white female	65 and over	.85	.96
Nonwhite male-nonwhite female	Under 15	.92	.98
Nonwhite male-nonwhite female	15–64	.75	.94
Nonwhite male-nonwhite female	65 and over	.97	.97
White male-nonwhite male	Under 15	.53	.67
White male-nonwhite male	15–64	.57	.35
White male-nonwhite male	65 and over	.43	.54
White female-nonwhite female	Under 15	.58	.66
White female-nonwhite female	15–64	−.60	−.43
White female-nonwhite female	65 and over	.72	.65
White male-nonwhite female	Under 15	.62	.70
White male-nonwhite female	15–64	.28	.24
White male-nonwhite female	65 and over	.33	.50
White female-nonwhite male	Under 15	.60	.62
White female-nonwhite male	15–64	−.17	−.24
White female-nonwhite male	65 and over	.75	.66

(continued)

NOTES TO TABLE 9-B-4

Note: Unlike the previous rates, the mortality data utilized in the table are age-adjusted by the *direct method,* using as the standard population the age distribution of the total population of the United States as enumerated in 1940. The change in the method of age adjustment was dictated by the time at which data became available and a desire to economize research resources rather than substantive considerations.

In order to ascertain whether the method of age adjustment and the use of data for nonwhites have important effects on spatial patterns in mortality rates, logarithmic regressions were run in which the dependent variables are the directly adjusted mortality rates for all ages while the independent variables are the previously utilized indirectly adjusted mortality rates for all ages. The results are shown below:

Group	Intercept	Elasticity	Coefficient of Correlation
White males	2.88	0.92	0.98
White females	2.85	0.97	0.98
Nonwhite males-black males	2.84	1.03	0.63
Nonwhite females-black females	2.82	1.64	0.89

The results suggest that the method of age adjustment does not make a great deal of difference for whites: the coefficients of correlation are very high and the elasticities are close to unity. As expected, the correlations between nonwhites and blacks are lower than those for whites but they are still fairly high, while the elasticity for males is close to unity and that for females between 1 and 2.

Source: *Mortality Data:* Mortimer Spiegelman, *Transactions of the Society of Actuaries,* 19, pp. D453–54, from tabulations made for the American Public Health Association under a grant from the United States Public Health Service (CH-00075).

Turning to spatial variability in mortality rates, coefficients of variation are observed to be greater for nonwhites than for whites within each age-sex group. For whites, female coefficients of variation are always higher than male coefficients; the same pattern exists with smaller relative differentials in the under-fifteen and fifteen to sixty-four age groups for nonwhites. However, in the sixty-five and over age group the direction of the sex differential is reversed—i.e., for nonwhites the male coefficient of variation is higher than the female coefficient. It is the above differences in magnitudes and directions which underlie the prior observation (Table 9–B-2) that for whites of all ages the female coefficient of variation is greater than that for males, while for blacks of all ages the male coefficient is slightly higher than that for females.[60] Patterns of spatial variability by age differ substantially

and that the age patterns of mortality of American Negroes ... differ from the mortality patterns of the white population of the United States."

[60] For some historical comparisons of male and female coefficients of variation,

according to race. For whites, the coefficient of variation is largest in the under-fifteen age group and smallest in the fifteen to sixty-four age groups; for nonwhites, variability is greatest in the fifteen to sixty-four group and smallest in the sixty-five and over group. It would seem that spatial differences in the factors affecting white mortality are smallest at working ages, while for nonwhites such differences are largest in this age group.

If a census division has a relatively high mortality rate for one age group, is it likely to have relatively high rates for the other age groups? Do the races and sexes differ in this respect? The most convenient way to deal with these questions is to convert the data into ranks and calculate the coefficients of concordance for each sex-race group. The latter statistic is a measure of agreement varying from 0 to 1 (representing perfect agreement among the ranks); its numerical value approximates the result which would be obtained by averaging all the relevant rank order correlations.[61] It is found that the probability that a census division having a high mortality rate for one age group will have relatively high rates for the other ages is somewhat greater for females and nonwhites than for males and whites. More importantly, the coefficients of concordance are quite low, ranging from 0.28 to 0.49. This strongly suggests that in future multivariate studies the results in the text that utilize mortality rates for all ages as the dependent variable should be checked by regressions utilizing age-specific mortality rates.

A visual examination of the ranked data reveals the following.[62] In the under-fifteen age group, the Mountain division is relatively high and the Northeast is relatively low for both sexes and races, while the Pacific is relatively low for nonwhites and the Mountain and East South Central divisions are relatively high for females. In the fifteen–sixty-four age group, the West North Central is relatively low for whites, the South Atlantic relatively high and the Pacific and Northeast relatively low for nonwhites, and the South Atlantic is relatively high for males. In the sixty-five and over age group, the Northeast is rela-

---

see Mortimer Spiegelman in the *Transactions of the Society of Actuaries*, 19, March 1968, p. D456. Spiegelman's evidence suggests that a reversal in the direction of the sex differential may have occurred.

[61] For a discussion of the coefficient of concordance, see Helen M. Walker and Joseph Lev, *Statistical Inference*, New York, Holt, Rinehart and Winston, Inc., 1953, pp. 282–86.

[62] In interpreting the results for nonwhites it must be remembered that there is a large Japanese population in the Pacific division.

tively high for both sexes and races, the Middle Atlantic is relatively high[63] and the West South Central relatively low for whites, while the West North Central is relatively high and the Mountain and Pacific divisions are relatively low for nonwhites, with the Mountain division relatively low for females. Perhaps the most interesting of the above findings is that the Northeast is especially favorable for the very young and especially unfavorable for the aged.

The data were next analyzed by means of the correlation techniques utilized for all ages; the results are collected in Table 9–B-4. The analysis of Table 9–B-2 reveals high positive correlations between the divisional mortality rates of males and females within both races. It is now seen that for whites the correlations in the fifteen–sixty-four age group are positive but quite low, which means that the high correlation for all ages is derived from the relationships in the youngest and oldest age groups. A similar pattern, although in a very much weaker form, appears for nonwhites. These results are not very surprising as sex differences in socioeconomic variables affecting mortality would be more pronounced in the fifteen–sixty-four group than in the younger and older groups. The correlation coefficients of Table 9–B-4 show that the previous finding of males of all ages being more highly correlated than females of all ages stems from a *negative* correlation between white females and nonwhite females in the fifteen–sixty-four age groups; the correlations for the other age groups are about the same for males and females. The inverse relationship for the fifteen–sixty-four age group is based on the fact that the mortality of nonwhite women is quite low in the Northeast and Middle Atlantic and high in the Southern divisions, while the reverse is true for white women. The unfavorable situation for nonwhite women in the South might be connected with childbearing, i.e., higher birth rates combined with less medical care, while Southern white women might be freer of pressures relating to work and earnings than Northern white women.

Returning to the question of a possible "reversal" of the socioeconomic roles of males and females in the black subculture, it is found that the evidence is inconclusive. If such a reversal actually occurred, it would be strongest in the fifteen–sixty-four age group, and, indeed, the correlation between white males and nonwhite females in this age group is positive while, as previously noted, the correlation between nonwhite females and white females is negative. At the same

[63] Mortimer Spiegelman has pointed out that in the Middle Atlantic the sixty-five and over age group contains a high proportion of the foreign-born.

time, the white male-nonwhite female and white female-nonwhite female correlations do not differ appreciably for the other two age groups. However, the reverse argument also suggests that nonwhite males, age fifteen–sixty-four, will have more in common with white females age fifteen–sixty-four than with white males of the same age, and this is not the case. The former correlation is negative while the latter is positive and relatively high. It must be concluded that no clear evidence of a reversal is provided by the more refined age-specific mortality correlations.

Index